THE INTEGRATED PRACTITIONER

Co-creating in Health Practice

BOOK 2 OF *THE INTEGRATED PRACTITIONER* SERIES

JUSTIN AMERY

Radcliffe Publishing
London • New York

Radcliffe Publishing Ltd
St Mark's House
Shepherdess Walk
London N1 7LH
United Kingdom

www.radcliffehealth.com

British Library Cataloguing in Publication Data

A catalogue record for this book is available from the British Library.

ISBN-13: 978 184619 774 1
Volume set ISBN-13: 978 184619 950 9

The paper used for the text pages of this book is FSC® certified. FSC (The Forest Stewardship Council®) is an international network to promote responsible management of the world's forests.

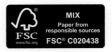

Typeset and designed by Darkriver Design, Auckland, New Zealand
Printed and bound by Hobbs the Printers, Totton, Hants, UK

Contents

Contents

These books are dedicated to my Dad, Tony Amery, who was a wonderful doctor and who is still my inspiration.

About the author

I am a full-time practising family practitioner and children's palliative care specialist doctor working in the UK. I have also spent some years working in Uganda and other sub-Saharan African countries.

I enjoy teaching, writing and mentoring. I am a medical student tutor at the University of Oxford, a trainer in general practice, and I have designed and set up children's palliative care courses for health professionals in the UK and Africa. I have worked with 'failing practices' to help them turn round; and also with health professionals who are struggling (as we all do from time to time).

I have always had an interest in philosophy and spirituality, and have studied this at postgraduate level. I have carried out some research into education and training of health professionals around the world and I continue to explore that interest.

I have previously written two books: *Children's Palliative Care in Africa* (Oxford: Oxford University Press, 2009) and the Association for Children's Palliative Care (ACT) *Handbook of Children's Palliative Care for GPs* (Bristol: ACT, 2011). I particularly enjoy reading and writing poetry.

At heart, though, I am a practitioner and a generalist. What is more, as you can probably see, I am rather a jack of all trades, and a master of none.

I have been motivated to write this book as I am hoping to explore practical ways of practising health that help us all, patients and practitioners alike, to become a little more healthy, and a little more whole.

Acknowledgements

These books have been brewing up over many years and so there have been very, very many influences upon them. There are far too many people to mention and thank without risking leaving someone out, so I shall just mention those who have been immediately involved.

Firstly, thank you to those very kind and patient people who helped review the drafts and gave such helpful feedback: Maria Ward, Penny Thompson, Meriel Lynch, Tom Nicholson-Lailey, Peter Burke, Penny Moore, Susan McCrae, Caitlin Chasser, Louise Rutter, Polly Steele, Rachel Samson, Laura Ingle and Maddy Podichetty.

I would also particularly like to mention Chris Smith, who not only gave very useful feedback on these books, but who also helped me to develop a lot of the ideas in them through his leadership of the Oxford Advanced Consultation Skills Course that I help him with, and over a few pints in the pub as well.

Thanks as well to Gillian Nineham of Radcliffe Publishing, who was brave (or daft) enough to put her faith in these rather unconventional offerings; suggest numerous areas for improvement and offer tremendous support and encouragement in their publication. Thanks also to Jamie Etherington and Camille Lowe for all their help in putting them together.

I would like to thank my colleagues at Bury Knowle Health Centre in Oxford, Helen House Hospice in Oxford, Hospice Africa in Kampala, Uganda, and Keech Hospice in Luton. They have all shown utmost patience and perseverance as I have led them on various merry dances, contortions and deviations in the name of 'good ideas', rarely reminding me of the 99% which failed, and always supportive of the 1% that, miraculously, did.

Of course I can't forget Karen Bateman (the doctor) and Karen Amery (the missus) who has been a continuous and never-ending source of sound advice, support and wisdom.

Finally, I would like to offer a huge thank you to Polly who, on a cliff top in Spain, gave me the courage to risk writing this stuff down and making it public.

Introduction to the series

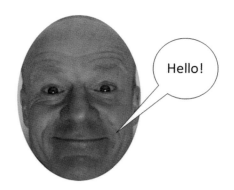

Hello!

Hello and welcome! This is me. You and I will be sharing a journey through this book, so you may wish to know what I look like. Because practice can't happen without practitioners, I will be popping up now and again, to test-drive some of the ideas that we will be discussing.

WHY ARE THESE WORKBOOKS NEEDED?

If you are, like me, a modern-day practitioner, you are probably still dedicated to the idea of good practice, but feeling rather buffeted by many and various winds of change that are sweeping through. You are also probably feeling (like me) that it would be good to have two minutes to sit back and reflect a little: to think about what's working and what's not; and maybe even to find a little balance.

If this is how you feel, you have come to the right place. So welcome!

In this series of workbooks we will be doing exactly that, taking a little time out, thinking about what we are doing, looking at things from different perspectives and using different lenses, and trying out some practical ways of making our practice more effective, more efficient, and (above all) more satisfying.

On the other hand . . .

If you are, like me, a modern-day practitioner, you will probably also be moving far too quickly to have any time for doing anything except what you need to be doing. In other words, you probably don't feel you have time for luxuries like sitting back and thinking. Frustrating though it may be, you probably have time to do only what you *have* to do, rather than what you *want* to do.

If this is how you feel, you are still in the right place, so welcome again!

In this series of workbooks, we will be working under the clock, recognising that there are boxes to tick and targets to hit. No doubt you don't just need to keep up to date, you need to prove you are keeping up to date too, for appraisal, or for review, or for revalidation. So, as we go along, we will be providing practical examples that will help you not just to reflect upon but actually to develop your practice.

What's more, we will even be providing appraisal certificates, so our appraisers, line managers and bosses will stay happy too!

> *But you're gonna have to serve somebody, yes indeed*
> *You're gonna have to serve somebody,*
> *Well, it may be the devil or it may be the Lord*
> *But you're gonna have to serve somebody.*
>
> — Bob Dylan

WHY DID I WRITE THEM?

I have written these workbooks because there doesn't seem to be anything out there that scratches my itch. Our experience of real-life health practice is messy, complex and often chaotic. It doesn't seem to bear much resemblance to the practice we read about, or even the practice we try to teach our students and trainees.

Modern scientific and philosophical understandings of the universe are complex, messy and relational too. But our models of health and health practice often seem to be built on glib and simplistic models, or they fall into dualistic discussions (for example, about 'patient-centred' or 'practitioner-centred' care; or about 'traditional' or 'alternative' practice; or even about 'disease' and 'health'). Is the world really like that?

I have also written these books as I am worried about the levels of demoralisation and burnout among students, trainees and colleagues that I meet, right across the globe. Of course we can all get a bit tired, burnt out, and maybe even ill. If we are honest, we are often sceptical and occasionally a little cynical about what we do. But if we are even more honest than that, at heart we believe in what we do, because we think it is important.

It's not that we want to turn the clock back. We can feel a considerable (if quiet) sense of pride in how far health practice has developed. But perhaps we'd also like to think that, in the 21st century, there is a way for our practice to include and yet somehow to transcend what has gone before. It's not that we want to reject the practicalities, the science, the technology and the politics. On the contrary, I think most of us wish to accept and value them. But we also want to do what evolution always does: including, building upon and then transcending what has gone before. In so doing, maybe we can also rediscover the art of what we do, and perhaps even find a way of expressing ourselves with a little more poetry.

WHAT WILL BE IN THEM?

The answer to that is simple really. We are hoping to look at practice from different perspectives, and using different lenses, so each book takes a different view.

- Workbook 1 – *Surviving and Thriving in Health Practice*. We are the foundation of everything we do. Without us there would be no health practice. We are our own most useful tools. So, in the first book, we will look at how we can keep ourselves sharp, surviving and thriving in practice.

- Workbook 2 – *Co-creating in Health Practice*. As practitioners, whenever we come into contact with our patients, we create something very familiar but also very strange: a relationship. This relationship is neither me nor the patient, but some sort of third entity, which has an existence of its own, partly from me, and partly from the patient. This 'co-creation' is arguably our most powerful tool, but it is a tricky one to use. So we will focus on that in the second workbook, considering how we might practise in a way that co-creates healthier and happier existences, for both our patients and ourselves.

- Workbook 3 – *Turning Tyrants into Tools in Health Practice*. As practitioners we have a vast array of tools that we can use: time, computers, money, information, colleagues, equipment, targets, our workplaces and so on. If they get out of balance, however, each of these tools can become a tyrant, so that it has control of us, rather than the other way round. So in workbook 3 we will be looking at some of the most important tools (and tyrants), considering how we can stay in control of them (and not vice versa).

- Workbook 4 – *Integrating Everything*. Health practice is, ultimately, a single integrated thing. While workbooks 1–3 have been looking at the different 'bits' of this 'whole', workbook 4 is where the rubber hits the road, because it is here that we try to put it all together and come up with ways that we can integrate everything into a happier, healthier and more skilful whole within the real-life, complex and messy world of health practice.

- Workbook 5 – *Food for Thought*. We are practitioners, so we are practical, and interested in practice. So we will leave the theory until last. But most of us like a little bit of theoretical background to give context to, and to underpin our practice.[1] So workbook 5 tries to provide that. Everything that exists does so against a background. Indeed the word 'exist' means to 'stand out'. All of our experiences, beliefs and understandings of health practice derive from a living, organic and constantly moving context: whether scientific, philosophical, cultural, aesthetic, biological or spiritual. It is useful therefore to spend a little time understanding and reflecting on these building blocks of who we are. As practitioners, we don't always have time to do this, so we will leave this book until last. It will be a little luxury for those with a little more time, not essential, but hopefully a bit nourishing. Like a fireside cup of cocoa.

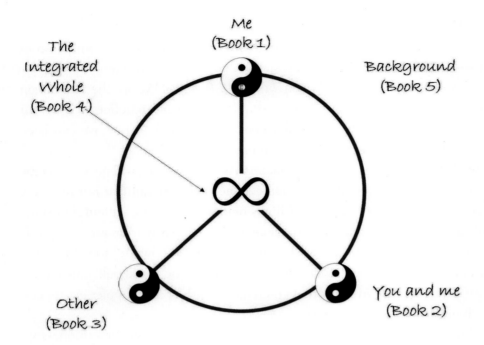

WHAT PERSPECTIVES AND APPROACHES WILL THEY USE?

In the 21st century we practise healthcare in a strange tension.

Science has taught us that we live in a highly relational, messy, multidimensional, complex, blurry and even chaotic universe. The humanities and philosophy have taught us that much of what we hold to be 'true' is relational and cultural and socially constructed. The arts teach us the value of creativity and expression in all walks of life. Spirituality teaches us about perspective, the value of awareness, and the fundamental interconnectedness of all things.

However, despite this relationality, creativity and complexity, we seem to be practising in a world that seems ever more bound and codified, with ever more targets and tick boxes, according to models that seem unrealistically geometric and two-dimensional, and with ever less room to breathe and to express ourselves.

So, in these workbooks, we will try to be practical and pragmatic. While we may not necessarily like the rules, regulations, guidelines, laws and targets that have nosed into our practice, we recognise that they have their uses. We know that health is a political football, and we are used to being kicked around a bit.

As practitioners in the 21st century we also value (and sometimes worry about) the advances that science and technology have brought. As practitioners, we are scientists, and we have a duty to do our best to ensure that what we do is as safe and effective as possible. We recognise that finding an evidence base for what we do is important not just for safety, but for development too.

So in these workbooks, we will start from the premise that we should, wherever possible, look for empirical evidence for what we are suggesting. On the other hand, we will remain vigilant to the blind spots of the empirical and technological approach, and look for alternatives to fill any gaps that we find.

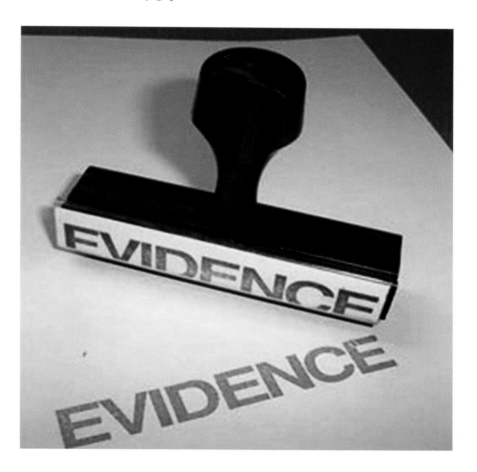

Wherever possible we will look for empirical evidence for what we are suggesting.

As modern practitioners we are scientists, and also technicians, but we are artists too. There is an art to being a practitioner, and in fact practice is an art. We might lose sight of it sometimes, but we are in the business (and busy-ness) of trying to create healthier and happier existences for our patients, and hopefully for ourselves too.

So in these workbooks we will be using plenty of imagery, art and illustration to engage the more creative sides of our brains, and to remind us that integrated practitioners need to be able to find balance between creative and practical.

These days, we don't tend to talk much about spirituality. Many of us would not think of ourselves as 'religious', and some of us might be horrified at the idea that modern-day practice should have anything to do with spirituality.

But most of us perhaps like to feel that there is some purpose or meaning behind what we do. We may hope that our practice connects with and somehow reflects the values and traditions of our families as well as of our broader societies and cultures. We deal with life and death, and so with the many existential and spiritual questions that arise as a consequence. If we are to be integrated practitioners, we need to have a handle on these too.

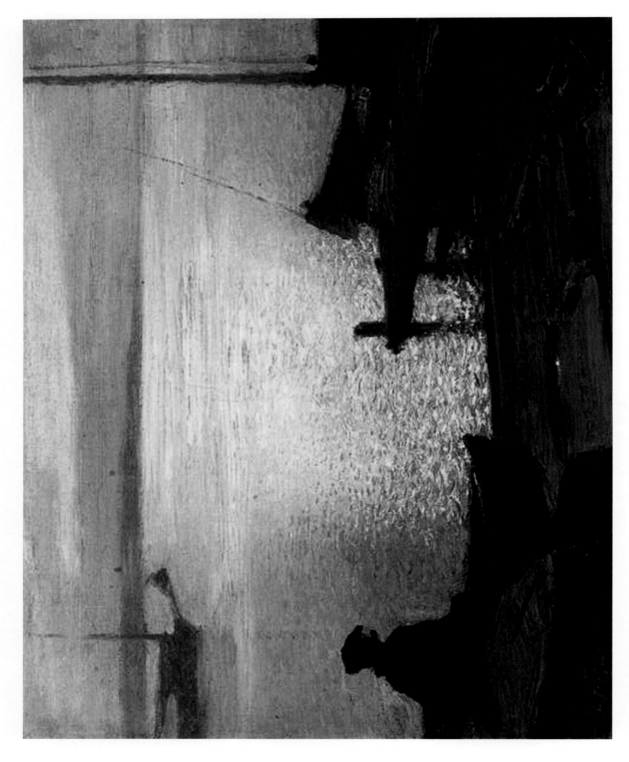

'Along the Mystic River' – for some reason I have found myself drawn to rivers as I have written this book, so a few will be popping up as we go along.[2]

So, in these workbooks we will try to look around the edges and to peer through the gaps, asking not just: 'What should we do?' but also 'Why should we do it?' and 'What does it all mean anyway?'

Finally, we don't have to practise long to realise that there are some things that make no sense, and from which no sense can be made. Random and chaotic events, reactions and emotions may arise, surprisingly. These can be both deeply troubling but also deeply wonderful, in that they can give expression to the inexpressible. We practitioners are practical people. We like to 'do' things. But sometimes there is nothing we can do, because there is nothing to be done. At these times, we have to just 'be'. For just 'being', for making sense of nonsense, and for making nonsense of sense, there is nothing better than poetry. So we will be seeing a fair bit of that too.

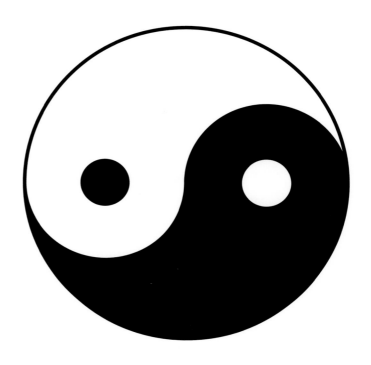

Symbols and rituals are fascinating things that in some way speak to us at a 'level beyond'. It is not often easy to make sense of them, and yet we may be surprised to find that our practice is full of them.

Ars Poetica

A poem should be palpable and mute
As a globed fruit,
Dumb
As old medallions to the thumb,
Silent as the sleeve-worn stone
Of casement ledges where the moss has grow —
A poem should be wordless
As the flight of birds.
*

A poem should be motionless in time
As the moon climbs,
Leaving, as the moon releases
Twig by twig the night-entangled trees,
Leaving, as the moon behind the winter leaves.
Memory by memory the mind—
A poem should be motionless in time
As the moon climbs.
*

A poem should be equal to:
Not true.
For all the history of grief
An empty doorway and a maple leaf.
For love
The leaning grasses and two lights above the sea—
A poem should not mean
But be.

— Archibald MacLeish[3]

POINTS AND PRIZES: SOMETHING FOR NOTHING

In the initial stages of this book, my publisher explained that medical publishing is at a turning point. Whereas before practitioners might choose a book that they would enjoy reading, nowadays they are too busy for that. So the upshot is that we only read books we need to read, rather than those we want to read.

A bit like Nanny McPhee...

The good news about adopting an integrated approach is we don't need to judge, we just need to adapt. If that is the way of the world, so be it, and so we have.

The particular way of the current world of health practice (at least where I currently work in the UK) appears to be a focus on objectives, outcomes, points and prizes. So the initial book has been adapted to match. Each chapter will contain activities and reflections that will meet common curriculum areas for medical and nursing practice. At the end of each book is a link to the Radcliffe Continuing Professional Development site, www.radcliffehealth.com/cpd, where you can download certificates that you can use for your CPD, appraisal or revalidation requirements.

OK, I admit it's a bit tongue in cheek, but there's no rule to say that we can't have fun while toeing the line, is there?

PROVISOS

I am, at heart, a practitioner, and a general practitioner at that. That means I am a bit of a jack of all trades, but master of none. I am partial, biased and subjective. The book is intended for all health practitioners but, inevitably, and despite my best efforts, no doubt the 'male', 'medical' and 'Western' nature of my experiences and thoughts will peep through. I hope you feel able to forgive them and look past them.

Also, I can quite honestly say that there is nothing new in this book, and I doubt there is anything in it that you could not find better argued and more coherently evidenced in other places. There is some philosophy, science, spirituality, art and poetry, but I am not a philosopher, scientist, guru, artist or poet. I am a health practitioner who dabbles.

So I have referenced those sources I can remember and can find. Others may be lost in the mists. But I do not claim any of the basic ideas in this book as my own. I have simply looked at them from my personal perspective and tried to put them together in a way that I have found useful in my own practice and in my own teaching. I hope you can enjoy them, and that you will forgive the numerous mistakes and omissions that you will undoubtedly find.

Chapter 1

Introduction to the 'we' relationship

Activity 1.1: Creation (30 minutes)

Find a flower. Look at it, touch it, smell it, feel it. Even shake it a little and listen to what you hear.

Now, take yourself back to your natural science lessons. How is your body sensing and perceiving the flower? Think, or note down, the different types of energy, force and mass that are in play.

Move forward, to your neurology lessons. What processes are going on in your nervous system that transmit and process the sensations that you receive from the flower?

Now, zoom out. See, feel, smell, touch and hear the flower again. Experience it with all of your consciousness. Does your description of energy, force, matter, electrical and chemical impulses adequately describe the depth and quality of what you are actually experiencing? If not, where is the 'existence' of this thing that you are holding? How does this 'existence' arise? Who makes it arise?

Reflect for a few minutes on the nature and properties of consciousness. Consider the possibility that you are creating what you are experiencing.

Consider the fact that you are experiencing yourself. Consider the even more strange possibility that you are creating yourself, and that we co-create each other.

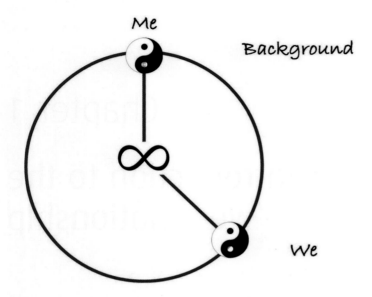

THE 'WE' CO-CREATION

We don't think of patients as our 'tools', but they are.

   Albeit a tool that is tricky to master . . .

As soon as we come into contact with another person, we co-create a new reality which is a product of both of us. That is, there is always a bit of me in what I see of you; and a bit of you in what I see in me.

   Everything we perceive is through the medium of our consciousness, and perceived by our consciousness, so we can *only* see that co-creation and the co-creation is *all* we can see.[4] As we will see in the following chapters, we start the co-creation automatically, the instant we meet, and that co-creation continues until we separate. Any boundaries that we perceive around the 'me' and the 'you' are much more leaky, blurry and fluid than we might think.

   What science and philosophy have taught us is that we are not disinterested observers on the 'outside' looking impassively and objectively 'in'. The co-creation *is* us at that moment. It is me expressing myself within you and within the universe; and it is the universe and you expressing yourselves within me; all together in one single, integrated whole.

   When we see our patients, one of the first things we do is to 'assess' them so that we can 'manage' them. However, the word 'assess', though deeply embedded in our psyche as health practitioners, is possibly distorting and hence problematic. The problem is that it suggests a one-way process between an impartial and objective 'assessor' and his or her 'subject'. As we have discussed, that is not how life is.

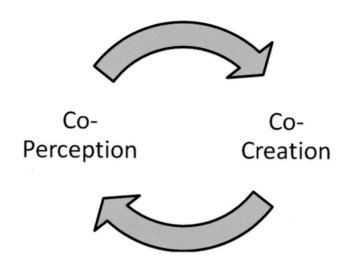

Co-Perception

Co-Creation

From our perceptions of mass, energy and forces in the universe around us, our consciousness creates the much richer 'existence' that we experience. When we are in relationship with another conscious being, we don't just 'create', we 'co-create', because both your and my consciousness are working in the same present. I perceive and create you as you perceive and create me, and we both perceive and create ourselves.

When two rivers merge, they automatically bring together and share everything with each other, for the moment they are together. They co-create one entity. That one entity can separate again, creating two more rivers. But then each river has changed, because each 'keeps' part of the other.

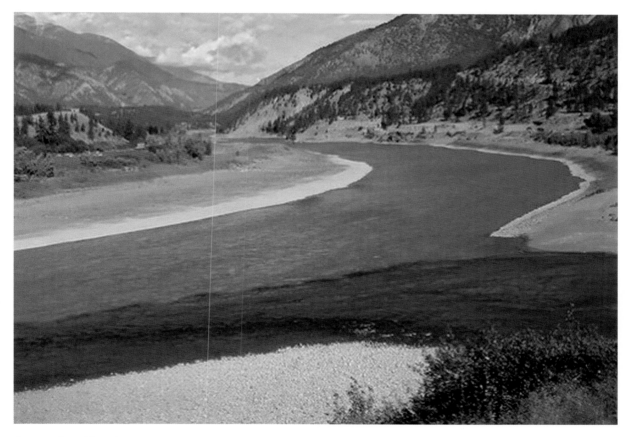

The merging of two rivers

COMMUNICATION

The way we co-create with each other is through the process of communication.[5] So this workbook will be all about how we communicate, how we co-create, as a tool for integrated practice. Health practice is beset by dualisms, such as health and illness, assessment and treatment, mental and physical, and so on.[6]

But that is not the way the universe is.

We exist at many different levels, not just two (for example, at atomic, cellular, personal and societal levels). So we can communicate at different levels.[7] As a consequence there are many different and sophisticated ways that we communicate with each other, and each chapter in this book will address a different level.

But in doing so we are not suggesting that these levels are inherently different things. They are all perspectives on the same, integrated whole; from the same, integrated whole.

Activity 1.2: Analyse your dualisms (30 minutes)

Health practice is full of dualisms, for example 'health' and 'illness'. These distinctions can be helpful as they give us systems for reducing, classifying, analysing, organising and practicing. But we don't exist in a reduced, classified or analysed world. Our world is also whole, messy and mysterious. As health practitioners we hope to be able to use both perspectives and many others too.

So spend a few minutes listing some of the dualisms that you currently use, and then consider how helpful each is in your day-to-day practice, and then how it may be unhelpful.

As practitioners, what we are looking for is perspective and insight into our fellow conscious beings, most particularly our patients. The clearer and more accurate this insight is, the clearer and more accurately we will be able to detect, discuss and amend their existences, and hence their health.

But that is not the whole story. Communication is two-way. By communicating 'right', we also give our patient a unique insight in what it is to be us. If what they experience through that insight is a practitioner who appears compassionate, courageous and honest, we have the best chance of our patients beginning to speak in an honest and forthright way, which gives us even further insight into them, and vice versa.

And if through our communication we feel better able to express and explore who we are, we may find that our health practice can also become a 'self-practice' in which we can create healthier existences for ourselves too.

At the heart of it all communication is the search for brighter light, for insight,

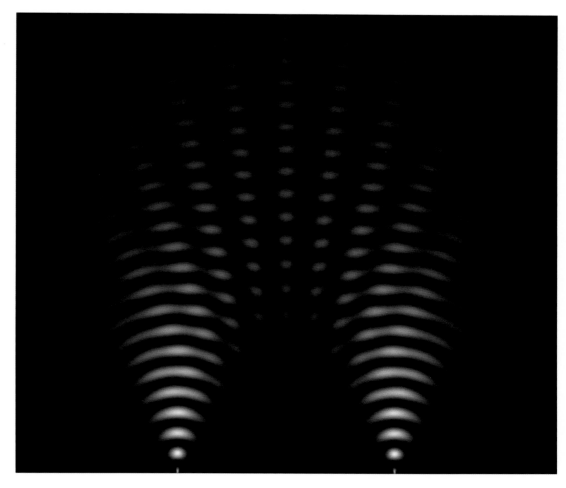

When waves from two light sources meet they 'interfere' with each other, creating peaks and troughs in that disturbance, which can be seen and measured. In the same way, when two (or more) people meet, the co-creation that they generate (through communication) is rarely smooth or harmonic. Using different communication techniques, we sense the similarities and differences between us; and then get drawn to explore and analyse these similarities and differences. Communication skills involve developing more subtle abilities to sense the disturbances and more effective abilities to communicate about them (without generating so much turbulence or dissonance that the relationship breaks down).

even for enlightenment. Insight illuminates darkness, listening fosters understanding, and speaking helps dispel the seeds of despair. That is the virtuous cycle that lies at the heart of effective practice.

> We don't think to ourselves: 'Ah! I have some visual and auditory information coming in. Let me consider how I put these together and compare it with my previous memories and ideas, and then paint myself an internal picture of my external existence.' We just see and hear, at one and the same time.

The Sounds of Silence

Hello darkness, my old friend,
I've come to talk with you again,
Because a vision softly creeping,
Left its seeds while I was sleeping,
And the vision that was planted in my brain
Still remains
Within the sound of silence.

In restless dreams I walked alone
Narrow streets of cobblestone,
'Neath the halo of a street lamp,
I turned my collar to the cold and damp
When my eyes were stabbed by the flash of a neon light
That split the night
And touched the sound of silence.

And in the naked light I saw
Ten thousand people, maybe more.
People talking without speaking,
People hearing without listening,
People writing songs that voices never share
And no one dared
Disturb the sound of silence.

'Fools' said I, 'You do not know
Silence like a cancer grows.
Hear my words that I might teach you,
Take my arms that I might reach you.'
But my words like silent raindrops fell,
And echoed
In the wells of silence.

And the people bowed and prayed
To the neon god they made.
And the sign flashed out its warning,
In the words that it was forming.
And the sign said: 'The words of the prophets are written on
  the subway walls
And tenement halls.'
And whisper'd in the sounds of silence.

— Simon and Garfunkel[8]

Chapter 2
Sensing

Activity 2.1: Spot diagnosis (1 hour)

Imagine you are Sherlock Holmes. Imagine that you are almost supernaturally alert; that you can see, hear, feel and smell even the smallest detail.

The next few times you meet a patient for the first time, be like Sherlock. Allow your senses to scan the patient and notice as many 'signs' as you can. Not just signs of 'disease' but signs of everything: of health, beliefs, culture, family, hopes, wishes. For each sign, interpret. What does it mean? What does it tell you?

Do it for a few patients, maybe five or ten.

Later on, when you have a bit more time, reflect on how many deductions you got 'right' or 'wrong'. Try to analyse what it was exactly that you sensed and how accurate you were at making deductions and interpretations based on the signs you sensed.

The basic building blocks of our co-creations are sense data.

Seeing, hearing, smelling, touching (and even tasting) are all crucial forms of communication in health practice. They give 'me' information about 'you', and vice versa. So our senses give us a huge amount of information with which we co-create each other and co-create health.[9]

We sense automatically, and often subconsciously. It is presumably a strong evolutionary advantage for us to be able to sense and act on information in the world around us as quickly and effectively as possible. Therefore, to some extent, we do not need to be trained to sense. It comes to us quickly, naturally and effortlessly.

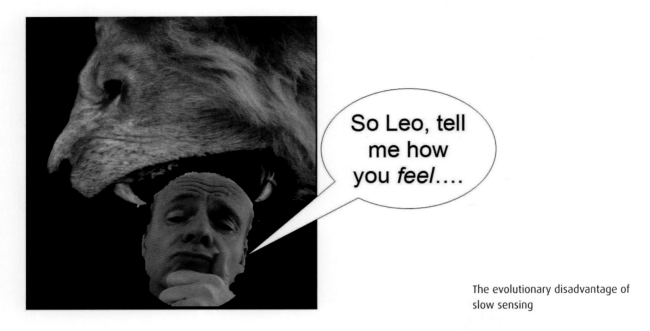

The evolutionary disadvantage of slow sensing

MEDICAL 'SIGNS'

Certain clusters of sensations occur together in ways that we are trained to look for. These clusters are known medically as 'signs'.[10] The general definition of signs is things that point to something else, but in health practice, we use the term more narrowly to describe exterior correlates of various states of health and existence.

Training helps us to use our natural senses to recognise clinical signs more skilfully. Furthermore, different types of practitioner are trained to sense different types of phenomena. For example, doctors and nurses may be trained to notice certain skin colours, heart and breath sounds, or normal and abnormal abdominal masses. A physiotherapist may be trained to notice certain musculoskeletal configurations, muscle tone, and stiffness of movement. A play therapist may be trained to watch for gross and fine motor movements, interaction behaviours, and forms of communication.

What is more, as we become more skilled and experienced, we begin to sense not just single signs, but patterns or clusters of signs ('spot diagnoses'). With training and experience, our recognition becomes so rapid and so subconscious that a 'spot diagnosis' may become intuitively evident even before we have said 'hello' to our patients.[11] We will explore the potential value of this learned intuition later in workbook 4.

But signs work both ways round. They say something both about the signifier and also about the signified. The 'signs' we choose to observe and ascribe meaning to are also signifiers of our personal perspectives, our underlying belief systems, our cultural narratives and our preferred forms of communication. Thus, to use them skilfully, we need to be aware of ourselves too, or we risk interpreting them through the distorted prism of our own prejudices.

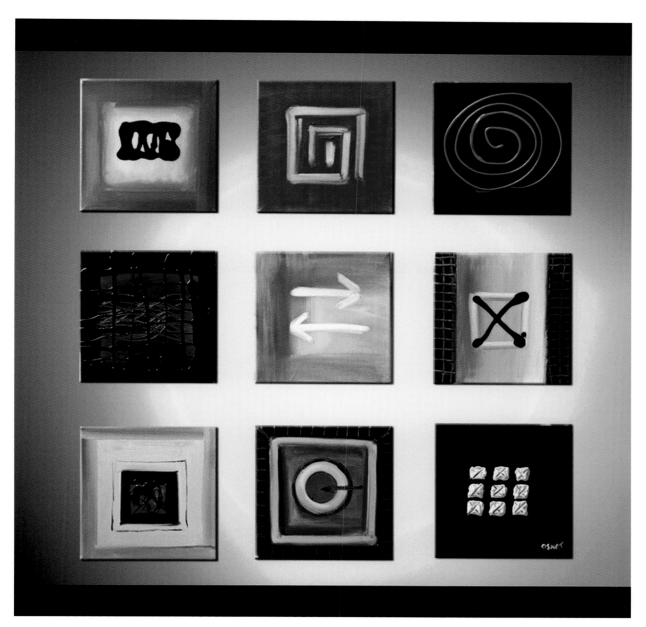

'Signs' – by Osnat Tzadok[12]

For example, a doctor may see a nosebleed as a possible sign of a clotting disorder, an allergist may see it as a sign of allergy, a counsellor as a sign of stress, and a traditional healer as a sign of spiritual possession. One sign, many meanings. So signs say almost as much about the signified as they say about the signifier.

Our senses are limited to relatively narrow spectra. Technology has made an enormous impact on health practice because it enables us to sense way beyond the limitations and bandwidth of our own sensory apparatus, thereby discovering a huge range of other physical 'signs'. Technology has also, through the development of computers, enabled us to interpret this data with ever more accuracy and speed.

It is difficult to believe now, but the technology on which we heavily depend is very recent. The stethoscope was invented just 200 years ago, X-rays were developed just over 100 years ago, and the sphygmomanometer even more recently than that. In the intervening period we have developed CT, MRI, nuclear resonance and ultrasound scanning; a vast range of biochemical, haematological, immunological and histopathological tests; the genome has been mapped; and we use microscopic surgical and optical fibre technology to observe and treat the body in ever more detail with ever less damage.

A wealth of signifiers. But what do they say about the signified?

INTERPRETING SIGNS

Sensing the data is only half the job. We have to interpret the data we sense so that we can draw conclusions that help us to make decisions and plans.

> Sensing and intuition describe the way we perceive, gather and interpret information. Initially we sense the data as raw data, then we try to match it to pre-existing cognitive scripts or patterns, and finally we attempt to make linkages between the information and other memorised or observed information. This final stage is what gives 'meaning' to the information.

According to the Myers-Briggs personality typology, we tend to have preferences either for sensing or intuition. In workbook 4, we will look at some of the limitations of thinking of sensing and intuition as opposites, but for now there is some value in thinking of them separately.

For example, those of us who prefer 'sensing'[13] may prefer to build the information carefully from the bottom up, arriving at meaning only once the foundations have been laid. Those of us who prefer 'intuition' may prefer to match and interpret data quickly, then use our senses to try to backfill and cross check the interpretation.

The risk of interpreting data without adequate sensing is that we may jump too early to conclusions. We therefore hope to be sufficiently systematic and thorough in finding data to support (or refute) our interpretations before we act on them. The risk of sensing without adequate interpretation is that we may fail to make relevant connections, or make them slowly or ineffectively. We therefore hope to practise and build from our experience in order to recognise patterns and linkages more quickly. So commonly, 'intuits' will accuse 'sensors' of 'paralysis by analysis', whereas 'sensors' will accuse 'intuits' of irresponsible leaps to unjustified conclusions!

In fact, both may be right, and we may be able to sense and jump to conclusions safely all at the same time, but we will explore that more in workbook 4.

Activity 2.2: Sensing or intuition (30 minutes)

Have a read through the poem below, and see what you derive from it. Then try to interrogate yourself to find out whether you tend to prefer 'sensing' or 'intuition' to assess new things.

The Whitewashed Wall

Why does she turn in that shy soft way
Whenever she stirs the fire,
And kiss to the chimney-corner wall,
As if entranced to admire
Its whitewashed bareness more than the sight
Of a rose in richest green?
I have known her long, but this raptured rite
I never before have seen.
– Well, once when her son cast his shadow there,
A friend took a pencil and drew him
Upon that flame-lit wall. And the lines
Had a lifelike semblance to him.
And there long stayed his familiar look;
But one day, ere she knew,
The whitener came to cleanse the nook,
And covered the face from view.
'Yes,' he said: 'My brush goes on with a rush,
And the draught is buried under;
When you have to whiten old cots and brighten,
What else can you do, I wonder?'
But she knows he's there. And when she yearns
For him, deep in the labouring night,
She sees him as close at hand, and turns
To him under his sheet of white.

— Thomas Hardy

THE UPSIDES AND DOWNSIDES OF SENSING IN HEALTH PRACTICE

The improvement in our ability to sense signs, either in person or using technology, has massively increased the range and scope of our health practice.

We can now diagnose, treat, screen for and prevent numerous problems that would have caused illness and death to our ancestors. Sensing in this way makes diagnosis more accurate, screening more specific, treatments better targeted and prevention more closely tailored to the needs of the individual patient.[14]

However, while there is little doubt that sensing as a form of communication has improved health and healthcare, we may also wish to take some cautionary notes, such as the following.

- Our objectivity may not be as objective as we think. 'I' cannot stand back, separate and distinct. When 'I' am with 'you', 'we' can only experience 'we'. Because none of us is perfectly self-aware, we cannot entirely differentiate between what we are sensing from another person and how our senses may be coloured or distorted by weaknesses in our sensing systems or by our own subconscious.

- Thinking of 'assessment' and 'treatment' as separate things may be to fall into a dualist trap. Assessment and treatment are contemporaneous, part and parcel of the whole process of co-creation. We may treat in assessing, and assess in treating.

- The way we choose to sense may affect what we find. The empirical approach and concurrent advances in technology have enabled us to be more scientific and systematic in how we 'assess', but it is still 'us' at the end point of the sensing process. By choosing to assess in one way or another (for example, choosing to use empirical rather than interpretive approaches) we influence what we co-create and so we influence what we experience of that co-creation. By choosing a hammer, we may turn our co-creation into a nail.

- Signs don't require our patients to say anything. Indeed, we have to ask our patients to be quiet and to keep still in order to discover many of them. As we have become more skilled at finding clinical signs, perhaps our patients have become more divorced from the process of health assessment?

- Technological sensing and treating requires technology, which means that patients have had to come out of their homes (and their cultures) into our practices and hospitals (and our cultures). Technology has also enabled us to sense signs that our patients cannot, and the significance of these signs has become increasingly divergent for ourselves and our patients. So perhaps medical 'signs' may signify not just 'disease', but also the dominance of a clinical narrative and increasing separation between practitioner and patient.

- We have started to pick up 'signs' not just of illness, but of potential illness. An example is high blood pressure. Patients do not feel ill if they have high blood pressure (unless it is extremely high). But when we diagnose people with hypertension, the evidence suggests that patients start to feel ill, and their quality of life deteriorates even though nothing has changed.[15]

- Finally, testing can be harmful.[16] The tests themselves can sometimes cause illness or death, false positive results can lead to unnecessary harmful treatments, wrong diagnosis can cause psychological distress; diagnostic labelling can cause stigma; and unnecessary or inaccurate tests can cause costs to both patient and society.

> The belief that a symptom is a subjective report of the patient, while a sign is something that the physician elicits, is a 20th-century product that contravenes the usage of two thousand years of medicine. In practice, now as always, the physician makes his judgments from the information that he gathers. The modern usage of signs and symptoms emphasizes merely the source of the information, which is not really too important. Far more important is the use that the information serves.[17]

INTEGRATING AND BALANCING OUR SENSES IN PRACTICE

As health practitioners, we are sensory beings, and our senses provide us with the core data that we need to co-create. With this core data we analyse, interpret, think, plan and then act for the benefit of our patients. Sensory data is therefore a core part of our co-creation with our patients. Without it, we will have an incomplete picture, and our actions will be less grounded.

Some of us may be brought up and trained in an empirical, medical 'paradigm' within which the primacy of sensing (particularly with technology) is now well established. Others of us may be brought up and trained within more cognitive, sociological, holistic or spiritual paradigms, and may distrust the role of sensing, and especially of technology.

As integrated practitioners, we hope to be able to take and keep our perspective. There are strengths and weaknesses of sensing, and technology has brought disadvantages along with its advantages. But few of us would refuse its benefits when we or our loved ones become sick.

Embracing the empirical and scientific approach does not have to conflict with values or ultimate beliefs. Like any other form of health practice it can be used compassionately, sensitively and effectively, for it is just a tool; and its inherent value lies with the motivation and skilfulness of the practitioner who applies that tool in practice.

Therefore, as we use sensory approaches, we hope to do so with mindful awareness, of ourselves, of others and of our machines. If the 20th century taught us anything, it is that machines can be truly wonderful, but they can also be truly awful. If we keep in mind the centrality of the patient in our practice, recognise the harms that a sensing approach can bring, and ensure we are as skilful as possible with their use, then sensing and technology can be extremely powerful tools in health practice.

But sensing and technology cannot take the place of communication, either conscious or unconscious, because it is through communication with our patients that we can learn and understand their values, ideas, concerns, hopes and wishes. Until we understand those, the sense data we received is much less useful, because we cannot interpret it or apply it in a way that is useful and meaningful for our patients, and thereby for ourselves.

Who Has Seen the Wind?

Who has seen the wind?
Neither I nor you:
But when the leaves hang trembling,
The wind is passing through.

Who has seen the wind?
Neither you nor I:
But when the trees bow down their heads,
The wind is passing by.

— Christina Rossetti

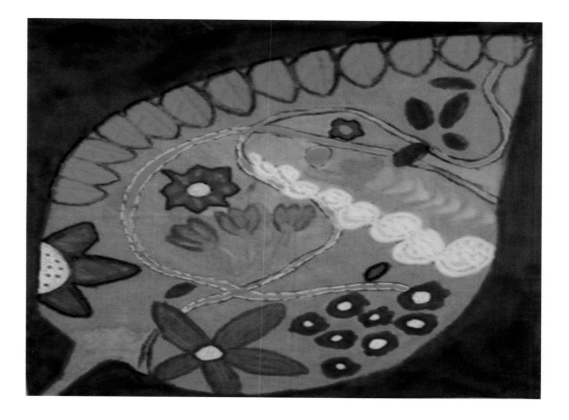

'Leaf' – by Mair

Chapter 3
Singing

At some point and for some reason, humans started co-creating each other by communicating through the expression of noises, rather like birds. Unlike birds, our song has become ever more complex and meaningful. So much so that we have stopped thinking of it as 'singing', and have got to know it better as speaking.

Which is a shame, as singing sounds so much nicer.

A WORD ABOUT WORDS

We live in an age where we have witnessed many amazing things. However, it is difficult to think of anything that is more amazing than the word. Because we are immersed in them all our lives, it may be that familiarity breeds, if not contempt, then at least disinterest. However, even a moment's thought (which we probably couldn't do without words) raises some fascinating questions about the apparently miraculous nature of them.

- What is meaning, and how can meaning, whatever it is, be expressed in sounds that I make?
- How on earth do my words mean anything to you?
- Does my mind create my words, or do my words create my mind?
- How is it that I can express the same meaning with different words, and different meanings with the same word?
- How can words make me cry, laugh, sing and shout?
- How is it that, through words, you and I together can create something that includes us, but is much bigger than the sum of us combined?

Kind words can be short and easy to speak but their echoes are endless.

— Mother Teresa

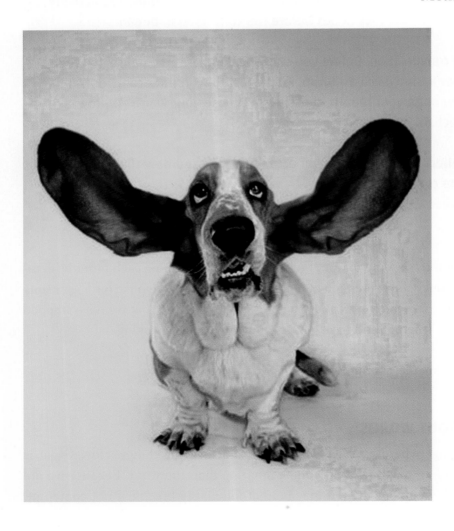

Big ears, small mouth . . .

That is not to say words are perfect. In many ways they are limiting. They are also difficult to use.

> We have less control over what we say and what we hear than we might think.[18]

Furthermore unskilful speaking or listening may make our patients less healthy, and may be unhealthy for us too.[19] However, there is little doubt that good verbal communication skills are important in health practice.

Before we go on to look at these skills in more detail, perhaps it is worth remembering the golden rule of good verbal communication. We can either hear or speak. It is difficult, maybe impossible, to do both effectively at the same time.

Words

Words are deeds. The words we hear
May revolutionize or rear
A mighty state. The words we read
May be a spiritual deed
Excelling any fleshly one,
As much as the celestial sun
Transcends a bonfire, made to throw
A light upon some raree-show.
A simple proverb tagged with rhyme
May colour half the course of time;
The pregnant saying of a sage
May influence every coming age;
A song in its effects may be
More glorious than Thermopylae,
And many a lay that schoolboys scan
A nobler feat than Inkerman.

– William Charles Wentworth

THE VALUE OF SILENCE

THE VALUE OF SILENCE

LISTENING

When we listen, we can listen in very different ways. We can arrange our features so it looks like we are listening, even though we are not. We can listen only in order to give ourselves a chance to rehearse what we want to say and then look for an opportunity to interrupt.[20] We can listen through a sieve, only listening for particular points of interest to ourselves. We can listen distractedly, wandering between listening to the other person and listening to our internal narratives.

Or we can listen deeply.

Deep listening[21] is listening not just to the content of the words, but also listening for the meaning behind the words, for the way the words are said, and for what is not said. It is a continuous and deliberate process of trying to build a picture of the whole person speaking and a picture of the whole context of the whole person speaking.

Deep listening is not passive, but it is active, conscious and poised. It uses body positioning, prompting, probing, use of open questions, non-verbal encouragement and verbal prompting to help our patients tell their story in rich and different ways, perhaps even in ways that they themselves were not aware of before the telling of it.

> I do not know if you have ever examined how you listen, it doesn't matter to what, whether to a bird, to the wind in the leaves, to the rushing waters or how you listen in a dialogue with yourself, to your conversation in various relationships with your intimate friends, your wife or your husband. If we try to listen we find it extraordinarily difficult, because we are always projecting our opinions and ideas, our prejudices, our background, our inclinations, our impulses. When they dominate, we hardly listen at all to what is being said. In that state there is no value at all. One listens, and therefore learns, only in a state of attention. In a state of silence in which this whole background is in abeyance, is quiet; then, it seems to me, it is possible to communicate.
>
> – Krisjnamurti, *Talks and Dialogues*

To listen deeply, we need to become aware of, and then consciously develop, our own inner silence. It is this silence which provides the pregnant, potential 'nothing' within which, and towards which, the speaker can express himself or herself, fully and completely as possible. And it is this silence, absent of anything, which enables us to listen and hear the co-creation that comes from our patients.

Deep listening is not just a useful tool for practitioners to hear and understand their patients. For some reason, simply listening in an empathic, unconditional, positive, non-judgemental way seems to be therapeutic just by itself.[22]

Cupboards

Drifting, dreaming
The door creaks open
Cupboardfuls tumbling
Onto the fleshly swept
Carefully kept
Floor
Rolling, rattling, unsettling

– JA

Activity 3.2: Deep listening (1 hour)

The next few times you meet a patient, be quiet. Not just that you won't speak much, but be physically quiet too. By all means make a polite greeting, but then sit back, disengage your mouth and engage your ears. Listen deeply. Don't interrupt. Don't even try to interpret. Just allow yourself to absorb everything that is coming from the patient – verbal and non-verbal. Don't panic if there is silence. Silence is golden, and its value will be returned to you in spades. So keep your breathing gentle, your muscles relaxed, and your mind clear. Gradually an image, or thought, or feeling will emerge. You will start to actually experience what it is like to be the patient, living with his or her problems. That's the mother lode. Now you can really start to practise.

RIGHT SPEAKING

No matter how respectful we are of silence, there comes a time in most communication when we have to speak. As practitioners we wish to be able to question, gather information, explain, teach, negotiate and plan with our patients. Unfortunately, the evidence about the effectiveness of our speech is not exactly good.[23]

Someone once said: 'A fool talks but a wise man speaks.' Whoever he was, I wish he hadn't, as those words are in my head now as a constant reminder of my status as the former. I also wish I had a pound for every time I have loosed off a volley of thoughtless, clumsy, daft, unkind or plain ignorant words.

Someone else once said, 'The easiest way to save face is to keep the lower half shut,' which is another bon mot I am trying harder to follow. In fact as I have got older, I have tended to speak less. I hope that I might fool others into believing that this is a sign of increasing maturity, but in fact it is simply that my memory is not what it used to be and I can't often remember what I wanted to say.

In practice we probably need to leave about a third of the time we spend with our patients on planning, educating and explaining. This is tricky, as it means we have less time than we think for listening, history-taking, cross-checking, examining and thinking. But there is a pay-off. The skills we use for right speaking and right listening are similar: openness, empathy, mindful awareness and imagination. If we use them effectively we will become more efficient (and more effective) at both listening and speaking.

Right speaking generally means thinking mindfully not just about 'what' to say, but also 'why' we want to say it. Asking this 'why?' question of ourselves before we speak helps us become more aware of the many, many voices in our internal dialogues; from there choosing the voice that will act most skilfully and compassionately in the current situation; and finally vetoing the voices that might speak out of other, less compassionate motivation.

In this way, we can think before we speak, and choose the apposite word at the opportune time.

PERSPECTIVE

Choosing the apposite word is not always easy. How do we know what will make sense to the patient?

One trick is to use the patient's own perspective. If we use our patient's own ideas, concerns, words and beliefs to communicate back to him what we want to say, he is most likely to understand and remember.

> In children's palliative care, we have to learn how to speak to children about very difficult subjects, for example about symptoms that they may suffer, or about death and dying. As adults, our normal reaction is to want to protect children from pain, so naturally we may avoid raising these difficult subjects. Unfortunately, the evidence is that children who are dying usually already know, well before their family or practitioners tell them. They often don't like to ask their parents, as they hate seeing their parents upset. So children can often get 'locked in' with their own questions and anxieties.
>
> We therefore try to train practitioners to be open to 'difficult discussions'. Often these discussions are fairly straightforward, because children are usually very direct and cut straight to the chase so, once the ice is broken, we simply have to answer their questions as they come up. There are well known pitfalls, however, and these come from our never-ending ability to pre-judge (wrongly) what the child is getting at.
>
> For example, I remember once speaking to a little girl who told me she

was scared of dying. I think I launched into a gabbling torrent of different reasons why she did not need to be scared. As I was holding forth I gradually came to realise that she was looking at me with that pitying, head-to-the-side, mouth-pursed look that my children get when they are thinking adults are being pretty dumb and in need of correction.

I backtracked rapidly and asked her why she was scared (which is how I should have started). It went something like this:

'Sorry. I think I'm missing the point?'

'Yes.'

'Right . . . OK . . . So, let's start again. You said you are scared of dying. Can I ask why? Are you scared of dying, or is it more that you are scared of being dead?'

'Oh, I'm not really scared of dying. It's more about what happens to me after I've died.'

'Ah. Are you worried about going to heaven or something?'

'No.'

'Oh. Are you worried about missing your family?'

'No. I know I will see them again in heaven.'

'OK. So what is it you are worried about?'

'I hate worms.'

'Pardon?'

'You know, worms. The ones that eat you when you are dead.'

'Ah. I see. (Long pause.) I'm not really sure what to say . . .'

'Well, can't I get a coffin that worms can't eat through?'

'Oh. Well, I don't know. But I'm sure I can find out. Was that all?'

'Yes.'

And off she went back to play (and I found a funeral director who could assure her that they could line the coffin so worms wouldn't eat through).

INTEGRATING SINGING INTO OUR PRACTICE

Sensing gives us hard data, which is crucial in health practice. Communication gives us perspective, because it puts that hard data into the context of what it is to be the patient, dealing with his problems, in her life. Without it, we cannot fully co-create.

From that perspective we can begin to see the value of skilful singing in practice. Right listening and speaking are not simply nice 'extras'. Failure to listen and speak effectively is highly unskilful in health practice.

We may therefore wish to dedicate and commit ourselves to learning and developing effective singing skills, whatever our practice or our specialty.

To sing well, we need to start right back at the background again. Right listening and speaking involve being mindfully aware of our own perspectives: of our values, beliefs, vocabulary, understandings, attitudes, prejudices and conceptions. It involves recognising that these will probably be different to those of our patients, so that, if we are unskilful with our communication, we will misunderstand each other. It is difficult to practise effectively from a foundation of misunderstanding.

As we have seen, words are almost miraculous. Through words we co-create a whole new existence that includes but transcends the 'me' and the 'you', the 'we' being greater than either. In this 'we' co-creation we don't just witness the existence of our partner, we experience that existence for ourselves.

By speaking and listening 'right', we can gain a unique insight into what it is to be our patient. As we will see later on, the quicker and better we can achieve that insight, the quicker, more accurate and more effective our practice is likely to be.

By speaking and listening 'right', we also give our patient a unique insight in what it is to be us. If what they experience through that insight is a practitioner who appears compassionate, courageous and honest, we have the best chance of our patients beginning to speak in an honest and forthright way, which gives us even further insight into them, and vice versa.

Song Unsung

The song that I came to sing remains unsung to this day.
I have spent my days in stringing and in unstringing my
 instrument.
The time has not come true, the words have not been rightly set;
only there is the agony of wishing in my heart.
The blossom has not opened; only the wind is sighing by.

— from *Gitanjali* (Rabindranath Tagore)

Chapter 4
Thinking, feeling and behaving

Activity 4.1: Vicious cycles (30 minutes)

Think of an aspect of your job which upsets you, or makes you anxious, or cross. Perhaps there is a certain patient or colleague, or a particular task, or a specific type of scenario. Sketch it out and describe it in some detail, either mentally or on paper.

Now sit back, allow your body to relax and your mind to clear. Address the scenario mindfully, and ask yourself the following question: Is the way you are thinking about this helpful or not helpful? For example:

- What automatic and unhelpful thoughts or conclusions does the scenario generate (such as 'Oh no, I'll never do this without losing it!')?
- Which of these thoughts or conclusions is 'hot' (in that it generates an emotional response (e.g. anger, fear, sadness)?
- How does the scenario make you behave? Which of these behaviours is unhelpful (e.g. avoidance, panic, anger)?

These are all characteristics of negative thought/emotion/behavioural loops, which infest health practice: both in patients and practitioners. But it doesn't have to be like this . . .

The life-blood of our co-creations are our thoughts, feelings and actions. Thoughts, feelings and actions are all highly relational, so by influencing one, we can influence the others. Words can directly influence all three, at the same moment.

So, for example, if you shout 'Watch out!' loudly to me, I will immediately stop what I am doing, my heart will race, I will feel anxious, I will rapidly think through what it might be I have to watch out for, I will try to locate it using all five senses, and then leap to avoid it. I will do this all at the same time.

HEALTH AS A CONCEPT, A FEELING AND A BEHAVIOUR

Health is a very desirable state of existence, yet it is also a very complex, all-embracing and hard-to-control state of existence. So, when we feel ill, we feel ill at many levels: cognitive, physical, emotional, psychological, social, behavioural, cultural and societal.

We think we are ill, we feel ill, we behave differently, and other people treat us differently.

Each of these is interconnected, so negativity in one can trigger negativity in all the others, and the overwhelming nature and breadth of this negative network can overwhelm our abilities to cope.

Words can help our patients by helping them break very big problems like this into smaller parts, and using our abilities to think and act rationally, to start to regain a sense of control and so a sense of health.

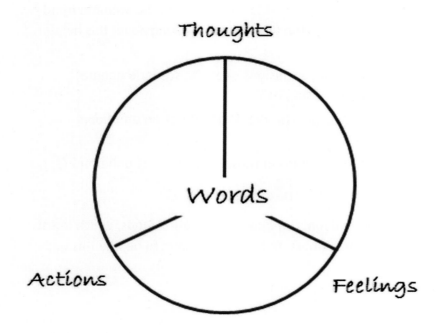

The influence and importance of words to how we feel, what we think and how we act.

For example, let's take a common scenario. Let's say we are tired, running behind and we've been interrupted for the fifth time that morning.

An unhelpful process might be:
- Thoughts: I can't believe it. Not again. Don't they know how busy I am? Nobody seems to care about me!
- Feelings: angry, sad, frustrated.
- Physical sensation: palpitations, chest pain, headache stiff neck, loose bowels.
- Action: shout at the interrupter.

Whereas a helpful process might be:
- Thoughts: Crikey, looks like everyone is having a busy morning. I'm tired, they are tired. We must try to grab some chocolate together later on.
- Feelings: tired and stressed but concerned for self and others.
- Physical sensation: tiredness, slight headache.
- Action: spend 5 minutes mid-morning with colleagues sharing a bar of chocolate.

Someone looking in from the outside can influence this whole chain of events simply by questioning the evidence for our initial assumption: in this case that *'nobody seems to care about me'*. If we can look for and discover evidence that in fact people do appear to care about me, and that they are not all out to get me, my mind, body and actions will be happier and more peaceful.

Both helpful and unhelpful cycles can become self-fulfilling. In the example above, if my actions include shouting at my colleagues, they probably will start to care less about me, and my suspicions will be confirmed, leading me to shout even more, and so on. If I share chocolate with them, they will probably care more (*or at least make me think they care more in order to get more chocolate next time*) and so I will feel happier, and more supported (*and more inclined to share chocolate . . .*).

Words can help us discover and break these vicious circles, both for ourselves and for our patients. When we can help ourselves and others see things more clearly, we can help to change things for the better – not just in theory but in practice.

We can use these 'cognitive' approaches (so called because they intervene at the level of cognitions, or thoughts) in many ways in order to help our patients, for example by doing the following.

- Being alert to vicious cycles of thinking, challenging them gently, and asking for evidence for different possibilities and perspectives.
- Asking our patients to recognise and keep notes or diaries of situations and events that trigger vicious thought cycles.
- Discussing negative and positive cycles and breaking these cycles down into manageable parts.
- Helping patients identify particular tendencies for unskilful thoughts, emotions, feelings or actions; and suggesting more skilful ones.
- Learning how to question unskilful or unhelpful thoughts and how to replace them with more helpful and more realistic ones.
- Discussing possible ideas and processes for changing unhelpful to helpful cycles.
- Practising them at home.

Activity 4.2: Helping patients stuck in negative thought loops (30 minutes)

If you have been in health practice more than a few days, you will have come across a number of patients who are stuck in negative thought loops. Think of one that you know quite well. Try to answer the following questions about that patient.

1. What negative thoughts does he/she hold about himself/herself? Can you think of any evidence against these negatives thoughts and conclusions?
2. Which of these thoughts is a 'hot thought' (i.e. it triggers a negative emotional response)? Can you help him or her learn and automate new and more positive emotional responses?
3. What behaviours does he/she act out that may make the spiral self-fulfilling? What alternative behaviours could you suggest and encourage?

Next time you see that patient, maybe you could try out some of your ideas.

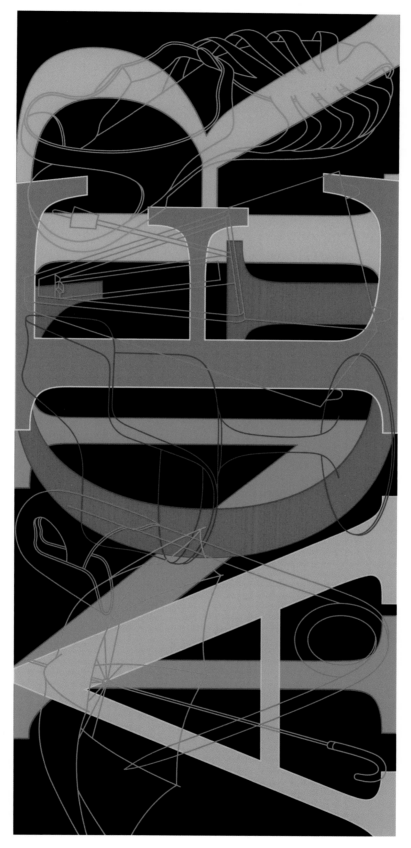

'Anger' – by Michael Craig-Martin.[24] Anger is a problem we all live with, as patients and as practitioners. But anger can be thought of as a 'secondary' emotion, often triggered by primary emotions such as fear or frustrated desire. It can also be a learned behaviour that triggers automatically in certain situations. Understanding our thoughts and behaviours like this can help us, and our patients, learn more effective and skilful patterns.

INTEGRATING COGNITIVE AND BEHAVIOURAL APPROACHES

In trying to develop healthy co-creations with our patients it is helpful to keep perspective of the mutual interconnectedness of thoughts, feelings and behaviours. Once we realise we can approach the same situation with different thoughts, different feelings and different behaviours we can see that we have a choice. We can choose to co-create using skilful and healthy cycles or we can choose to co-create using unskilful, less healthy ones.

As practitioners of almost any type, these 'cognitive' and 'behavioural' approaches to practice can be highly valuable, as they can be used in almost any context (please see the endnotes for more information[25]).

By communicating effectively with our patients we can listen out for, and become mindfully aware of, unskilful thought cycles that our patients (and ourselves) may have slipped into. Once we are aware of them, we can start to question, dissect and analyse them, to identify unhelpful or illogical assumptions or steps; and to suggest more helpful and more logical alternatives.

This comes together as a very neat, effective, and quite quick intervention that has many uses and many applications in health practice. Because it is quick and effective, it is usually a tool we can integrate fairly readily into our practice, whatever that practice is.

My Soul is Dark

My soul is dark – Oh! quickly string
The harp I yet can brook to hear;
And let thy gentle fingers fling
Its melting murmurs o'er mine ear.
If in this heart a hope be dear,
That sound shall charm it forth again:
If in these eyes there lurk a tear,
'Twill flow, and cease to burn my brain.

But bid the strain be wild and deep,
Nor let thy notes of joy be first:
I tell thee, minstrel, I must weep,
Or else this heavy heart will burst;
For it hath been by sorrow nursed,
And ached in sleepless silence, long;
And now 'tis doomed to know the worst,
And break at once – or yield to song.

– Lord Byron

Chapter 5
Storytelling

Activity 5.1: Stories of you (1 hour)

Describe yourself in one paragraph. Write it down so you can go back and look at the words and phrases that you have used. Now describe yourself as a close family member or friend would. Finally, describe yourself as your patient would.

Look at the three descriptions: particularly the nouns, adjectives and adverbs. Consider how the three 'narratives' about you are similar and how they differ. Which is 'true'?

We all love a good story, particularly when we are in it.

A wonderful but also very useful perspective is to see our existences as co-creations woven from the interplay of many different stories. These are stories that we tell ourselves, each other, and our world; about ourselves, each other and our world. It is partly through the telling and retelling of these stories that our lives derive meaning and purpose.

So narratives are the stories we tell ourselves and each other,[26] but they are also more than that. They are intricately tied up in our sense of personal identity, and in some ways our narratives *are* who we are.

Our patients may come to us because they have told themselves (and been told) particular stories about their health that lead them to decide they are unwell, and that in turn leads them to our door. As we have seen in this series of books, ill health means different things to different people, so unless we understand their stories, we cannot fully understand how we can help our patients in a way that is meaningful to them.

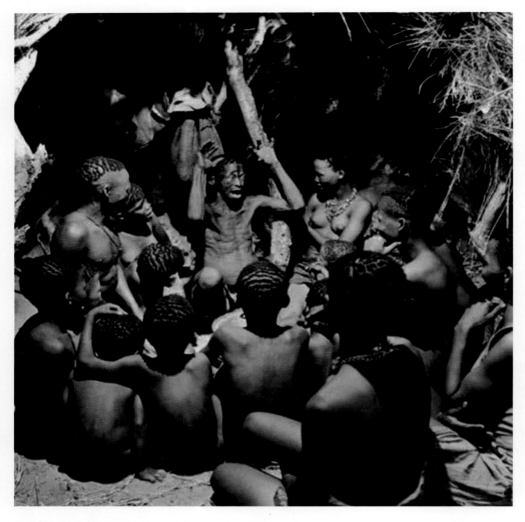

'A tribal chief acts out a story to children in the Kalahari'.[27] Through stories people learn about their history, their identity, their aspirations, their relationships – in short, their identity.

THE ESSENCE OF STORYTELLING

The words 'narrative therapy' may sound grand, even off-putting. But if we think of it simply as storytelling, it becomes much more accessible and easier to understand.

We all know what makes a good story: an interesting plot, fascinating themes, rich and complex characters, evocative imagery, and choices of words and phrases that suit the nature of the story. Good writers look for all of these, and a good story feels rich and believable. Bad writers miss the mark, and can leave us with stories or characters that are thin, flat and unbelievable.

Activity 5.2: Imagery (30 minutes)

As an illustration of how words, metaphor, characterisation and plot influence the narrative, consider the three poems below: one from 18th-century Scotland, one from 20th-century Australia, and one from 7th-century Japan. See how the combination of words, sounds, characters, plots and images create quite different narratives, which are so effective we can almost 'be there' in the completely different worlds and existences that the poets create.

From Tam o'Shanter

When chapmen[1] billies leave the street,
And drouthy[2] neibors, neibors, meet;
As market days are wearing late,
And folk begin to tak the gate,
While we sit bousing at the nappy,[3]
An' getting fou[4] and unco happy,
We think na on the lang Scots miles,
The mosses,[5] waters, slaps and stiles,
That lie between us and our hame,
Where sits our sulky, sullen dame,
Gathering her brows like gathering storm,
Nursing her wrath to keep it warm.

[1 Hawker; 2 Thirsty; 3 Beer; 4 Drunk; 5 Marshes.]

— Robert Burns

Then and Now

No more woomera, no more boomerang,

No more playabout, no more the old ways.

Children of nature we were then,

No clocks hurrying crowds to toil.

Now I am civilized and work in the white way,

Now I have dress, now I have shoes:

'Isn't she lucky to have a good job!'

Better when I had only a dillybag.

Better when I had nothing but happiness.

— Oodgeroo of the tribe Noonuccal[28]

Autumn day viewing Shinsen'en Garden

Step with the left foot, step with the right foot, Shinsen
 seasonal things.

Mind confused cannot return.

High terrace god reached with non-human power.

Pond mirror clear deep pool containing radiant sunshine.

Crane sound reverberates heaven, tame in the imperial
 garden.

The snow-goose wings hesitate, folded up about to fly.

Swimming fish frolic in seaweed, their fate to swallow a
 hook.

Deer call, deep grass dew dampened clothes.

All that roam all abide, feeling the sovereign's virtue.

Autumn moon, autumn wind, the entry doors of emptiness
 (Sunyata).

Holding grass in their mouths, chewing the bridge to what
 non-existence?

Patter, patter, leading one another in dancing the profound
 mystery of existence.

—Kukai

NARRATIVE THERAPY

Sometimes, we tell ourselves stories that are unhelpful. For example, we may tell ourselves stories in which we are helpless, or hopeless, or useless, or bad, or sick, or mad. Sometimes, these 'unhelpful' stories can become tyrannical, blotting out all other stories about ourselves, so that we begin to 'believe' in the negative characterisations of ourselves (for example, that we are 'helpless', 'hopeless' or 'useless'). When particular narratives and characterisations become tyrannical, they dominate our sense of self, thereby rendering us 'unhealthy'.

As practitioners, if we can begin to recognise these unhelpful stories and characterisations, we can work with our patients to try to find new and healthier ones. We can do this by employing all the tools we would use to write any story: plot, characterisation, words, metaphor, theme, tempo, setting and sequence.[29]

> So, for example, I have recently been seeing a patient who says that that she is 'exhausted from constantly swimming against the tide of bad luck'; and she now feels that she is 'drowning under a relentless flood of stresses and upsets'.
>
> In that kind of statement we can clearly see plot (e.g. woman gradually drowns), metaphor (e.g. flood, drown, swim, tide), tempo (e.g. slow, relentless exhaustion), characterisation (e.g. helpless 'her', remorseless 'bad luck'), theme (e.g. hopelessness and helplessness of mortals in the face of overpowering external forces).

As our patients tell us their stories, so we can help them to identify and recognise them as stories. What's more, see them as stories that they and those around them have authored (or co-created). Once they recognise and identify a particular story, we can help them to bring it out into the light, and look at it as a critic might look at a novel.

Our role in this is not to get the patient to choose one story over another, but rather to help the patient to act as an 'investigative reporter', to disentangle their narrative from their internal world, 'externalise' it, deconstruct and analyse it, and then reconstruct it into a narrative that is richer, more whole, and more healthy.[30]

The key theme behind narrative therapy is that 'the person is not the problem'. By helping a patient externalise a problem, we can help him separate his identity from his harmful narratives. In this way, perhaps he can begin to draw out some alternative stories that, however 'thin' they are compared to the richness of the dominant story, are still stories that are sensible and meaningful for him. It is not that we decide which story is good or bad for our patient, it is that we help him see that the he already has alternative stories, and that he can choose one or more of them to tell, and so to create and to live.

This is a lot of jargon, but the idea is not complicated. The point is that we weave our stories into our internal thoughts and ideas, so that it becomes difficult to work out where the story stops and we begin. Rather than us creating our stories, our stories begin to create us. By getting patients to talk about their stories, we help them realise that their stories, and so their existences, can be changed.

From there it becomes a question of helping our patients to act as authors in the new stories they wish to tell. Initially, these new stories may be very 'thin' and weak. However, with help, they can add complexity, colour, texture and richness, so that the new healthier story becomes more dominant, and the unhealthier ones recede.

So in my example of the 'drowning patient' above, we might wish to point out and gently challenge the metaphors and imagery she is using, and check to see if the story we are hearing is the same as the one she is telling. We could ask our patient to identify her two characters – let's call them 'little Miss Helpless' and the evil 'Count Remorseless Bad-Luck' – and then 'bring them out of her subconscious and into the light (externalisation). Once they are out, we can sit them down next to us and cross-examine them. So, for example, she might ask the evil Count: 'When did you start dominating little Miss Helpless? Can you dominate her all the time? Is there ever a time or place where you are less certain of your dominance, and another character (say Sir Galahad Good-Luck) has ridden over the crest of the hill?' Or she might ask Little Miss Helpless: 'Was there ever a time you didn't feel helpless? Is there any way you might benefit from being helpless? Who around you helps you to feel more in control? Are there situations where you feel you might in fact be able to free yourself from the Count?'

While we may not be able to bring all of the skills and time that a narrative therapist may, narrative approaches still offer us many techniques that we can weave easily into our everyday practice, for example the following:

- Looking for internalisations: e.g. 'I am a worthless person', 'It's my optimism that got me through'.
- Looking for thin descriptions: e.g. 'I am an attention seeker', 'an alcoholic', 'an abuser'.
- Looking for thin conclusions: e.g. 'So I will always be a drinker', 'an abuser', 'an attention seeker'.
- Changing the adjectives that people use to describe themselves into personal nouns: e.g. if someone says 'I am a depressed person' we may ask 'How long has this "depression" been influencing you?' or 'What does the "depression" tell you about yourself?'
- Once externalised, putting problems into storylines: e.g. how long the depression

has been an influence, when it came, factors that contributed to its entry, its real effects, when these effects have been strongest and weakest, what sustains it, what remedies its effects.

- Using real not given names: e.g. not 'anxiety' but 'the fear, the panic, the wobbles, the shakes'.
- Using personification to reduce power of words: e.g. Mr Diabetes, Ms Fear.
- Bringing in new more supportive characters: e.g. Mrs Supportive.
- Watching metaphors carefully: e.g. trying to change combat, conflict or violent metaphors to more hopeful, gentle and compassionate metaphors.
- Looking for unique outcomes: e.g. times when the patient has been free of the problem. Then exploring what, when, who, how that happened.
- Intervening occasionally: Encouraging patients to talk to witnesses who have seen their more positive states, or to write therapeutic letters or diaries for themselves, or to use rituals and celebrations to cement in healthier narratives.

Activity 5.3: Using narrative in practice (1 day)

For the next few patients you see, keep a notebook handy. Write down any interesting verbs, nouns, adjectives, adverbs or metaphors they use to describe themselves and their life.

As you get more confident, try taking on the role of 'investigative reporter', seeking out and exposing negative or 'thin' stories. To start with, just reflect them back to the patient. Later, try helping the patient start to tell more helpful stories about themselves, using more positive imagery, and always seeking happier endings.

INTEGRATING NARRATIVE INTO OUR PRACTICE

Initially, it may seem odd to think ourselves as the co-creations of stories, rather than the other way round. However, a little reflection suggests that there was never a time, at least outside the womb, that we weren't in the midst of, authors of, subjects of, listeners to and tellers of stories about ourselves, our families, our peer groups and our cultures. From this perspective we can 'zoom out' and start to look at ourselves and our practice afresh. What are the stories that we have been told, and that we tell ourselves, which underpin who we are, what we are and where we are?

As we think about our narratives, we will start to identify certain stories about ourselves that are supportive and creative; and others that are undermining and destructive. We don't have to value all our stories equally. It is a matter of choice which ones to believe and which ones to act out.

This kind of perspective may help us to become more mindfully aware of those stories that we use within our own lives and our own practice; and which ones may be more or less helpful with various different patients.

As we become aware, we realise that we have the ability to use stories to re-create healthier co-creations with our patients, We can choose which stories we wish to change, or to retell, or to cast out altogether. Those we value we can enrich and thicken by moulding the words, plots, characterisation and imagery by thinking and talking about them. And those which are useful we can begin to incorporate into our own practice, so that our stories begin to interweave with the stories of our patients, taking care to author them in a way that leads us both to a healthier, more integrated and harmonically balanced outcome.

The Thin People

They are always with us, the thin people
Meagre of dimension as the gray people

On a movie-screen. They
Are unreal, we say:

It was only in a movie, it was only
In a war making evil headlines when we

Were small that they famished and
Grew so lean and would not round

Out their stalky limbs again though peace
Plumped the bellies of the mice

Under the meanest table.
It was during the long hunger-battle

They found their talent to persevere
In thinness, to come, later,

Into our bad dreams, their menace
Not guns, not abuses,

But a thin silence.
Wrapped in flea-ridded donkey skins,

Empty of complaint, forever
Drinking vinegar from tin cups: they wore

The insufferable nimbus of the lot-drawn
Scapegoat. But so thin,

So weedy a race could not remain in dreams,
Could not remain outlandish victims

In the contracted country of the head

Any more than the old woman in her mud hut could

Keep from cutting fat meat
Out of the side of the generous moon when it

Set foot nightly in her yard
Until her knife had pared

The moon to a rind of little light.
Now the thin people do not obliterate

Themselves as the dawn
Grayness blues, reddens, and the outline

Of the world comes clear and fills with colour.
They persist in the sunlit room: the wallpaper

Frieze of cabbage-roses and cornflowers pales
Under their thin-lipped smiles,

Their withering kingship.
How they prop each other up!

We own no wilderness rich and deep enough
For stronghold against their stiff

Battalions. See, how the tree boles flatten
And lose their good browns

If the thin people simply stand in the forest,
Making the world go thin as a wasp's nest

And grayer; not even moving their bones.

– Sylvia Plath[31]

Chapter 6
Hypnotising

Activity 6.1: Self-hypnosis (30 minutes)

- Get into a comfortable position.
- State your purpose for the session: e.g. 'I'm going to try self-hypnosis to try to improve my health practice.'
- Relax your body using progressive muscular relaxation, gentle breathing, or by imagining waves of relaxation course through your body, washing out any tension.
- Deepen your relaxation by imagining your thoughts and emotions drifting away like clouds, or go back to a pleasant memory of a relaxing time, and try to visualise it very clearly.
- Now allow your attention to turn to yourself. Visualise yourself as an excellent practitioner in practice.
- Ensure all your senses are engaged: what can you see, feel, hear and smell? Don't get drawn into thinking or analysing. Just watch. If emotions or thoughts arise, just smile at them and allow them to drift off. Spend a few minutes peacefully watching yourself practise excellently.
- Consciously come back to yourself, allow your eyes to open and become aware of the room around you.
- Vocalise or write down any ideas or plans that have arisen.

As we go about creating ourselves, every now and again, we find ourselves completely absorbed in the moment, and so focused on what we are doing that everything else disappears from our mind.

At those moments we seem to have complete clarity.

Sometimes these moments arise out of an unpleasant experience, such as an accident. Sometimes, they arise out of moments of deep joy, such as the birth of a child. But they can happen at more mundane times too: perhaps when we are absorbed in a good book, or out on a walk, or even just watching our children play.

USEFULNESS

These moments of absorption and clarity are sometimes referred to as trances. Trances are highly focused and aware states of mind.[32] They are also states of mind that are highly suggestible, as they are states in which our psychological defences are temporarily down.

Trances are therefore states of mind that can be very useful in health practice, particularly when we are trying to help patients come to terms with a new idea, deal with the anxiety and stress of physically or emotionally painful events, face up to a new reality, or change behaviours in some way.[33]

Unless we are trained and practised in hypnosis, and have the time and resources to carry out full sessions, it will be difficult for most of us to use hypnosis systematically. But the essence of hypnosis is straightforward and common sense: relax, think positively, visualise what you hope to achieve (or to stop), meet and deal with emotions that arise, and then try to learn and anchor more effective and more 'healthy' behaviours.

These are all things that we commonly try to achieve with our patients from time to time

It may therefore be useful for us to be aware of the potential benefits of trance induction, of how we might induce brief trances, of ways in which our patients may use them[34] in order to become more aware of ill health, more focused on healthy behaviours, and more suggestible to healthy changes.[35]

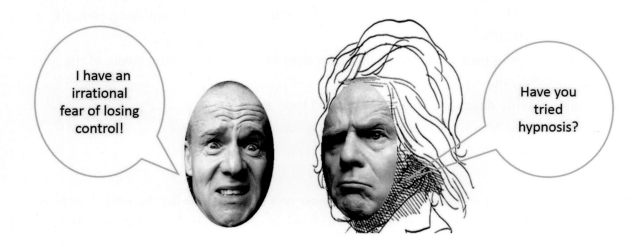

Hypnosis – with apologies to Doug Savage

PREPARATION

Hypnosis, like mindfulness, requires that we are at ease, relaxed and fully focused in the moment. To try to help our patients into this state, there are a few simple things we can do.

- General warmth, friendliness and politeness of greeting.
- Gentle touch early on, for example with a handshake (where acceptable).
- Creation of a 'neutral' environment, within which patients can express themselves (rather be dominated by the expression of the practitioner's own identity into the space).
- Use of gentle and peaceful silence at the beginning of a consultation.
- Use of tones and qualities of voice that are calming.
- Use of calm and peaceful body language.

INDUCTION

With more time available to them, hypnotherapists may use a variety of techniques to relax their patients further, for example by using progressive muscular relaxation, calming monologues, or through getting the patient to visualise desired outcomes. The idea is that, as we become more relaxed, we become more suggestible and more able to access thoughts or ideas that might be normally difficult for us to access.

In general health practice, it is unlikely we will have the time or skill to do all of this fully. However, there are brief hypnotic interventions that we can learn and use, derived from Eriksonian[36] hypnosis techniques. Being simple and quick to use, they are eminently suitable for everyday health practice.

These techniques aim at trying to induce or guide patients quickly into particular states of communication, thought or action, and they include the following.

- Inducing positive self-belief with 'generalisations' and 'deletions': *e.g. 'I'm always amazed by how well you cope.'*
- Just before we want to make a suggestion, or in order to change patients away from unhelpful patterns of speech and behaviour, we can generate brief moments of cognitive dissonance, and hence momentary trance, in our patients' minds by (for example):
  - using deletions in our speech: *e.g. 'Well, I just wonder if . . . maybe not . . . but . . . perhaps you might feel better if you lose some weight'*
  - using touch or changes in body posture to distract patients when they are using unhelpful patterns of speech, or just before we want to make a suggestion, *e.g. moving forward, or suddenly looking up, sighing, stretching*
  - leaving gaps in our speech or our actions: *e.g. 'I have always been amazed by how well you seem to . . ., well, you know what I mean!'*
- Making subtle suggestions: either directly (*e.g. 'You clearly care about your fitness'*) or indirectly: *'I wonder if you are aware of how much more you care about your fitness than some of my other patients.'*

- Telling stories as metaphors for our patients' own situation: *'Do you know, I once had a patient who had a terrible time. Lost his wife to cancer you see. He almost went under, what with his drinking and everything. He didn't think he would ever be able to stop, and to be honest nor did I. It wasn't easy, and it took him a few goes, but he managed to get dry in the end.'*
- Embed commands by using certain entry phrases, dressed up as an observation or question: For example:
  - *'What would it be like if you were to* **stop smoking***?'*
  - *'If you were to think that you could* **sort out your relationship***, I wonder if you would feel compelled to* **act on it.***'*
  - *'I wouldn't feel at all surprised if you were to* **do some more exercise***, as I have always found you to* **be very resourceful.***'*
- Use 'process instructions' which draw upon a patient's memories or experiences from the past and direct them to applying that to a new situation. A simple example would be: *'I was hoping to check your blood pressure, and while I do so it might be very helpful if you could take yourself back to a warm, sunny beach where you felt so relaxed and peaceful.'*

ANCHORING

Once we have raised particular helpful suggestions, we can help our patients fix these suggestions in their minds using a process called 'anchoring'.[37] Anchors are automatic associations between a stimulus and our response. We all have them.

> For example, we may find we lose our temper easily when we are cut off by another car, or we might be instantly taken back to a schoolroom by the smell of a certain floor polish, or we might feel a sense of exhilaration when we see a beautiful sunset.

They are presumably evolutionary or adaptive response 'short circuits' that we have learned in order to act quickly in the face of certain situations. In health practice we may come across them in severe forms when our patients come with phobias, or post-traumatic flashbacks. However, they can occur in simple and less extreme ways, for example 'white coat' hypertension, waiting room anxiety or even perhaps the placebo effect.

As they are learned responses they can be shifted and anchored to other, more pleasant responses.

> So, for example, we might teach ourselves to sing the Marseillaise rather than make offensive gestures every time we get cut off by a car (although there is a downside – we might then think about bad drivers every time we hear the Marseillaise!)

In health practice we can help our patients to discover and explore unhelpful anchors; and help them form more positive associations, without trying necessarily to analyse or explore what might be behind them. In that way anchoring is a form of behavioural therapy. In ordinary health practice it is unlikely we will have sufficient time to carry out full behavioural therapy in patients with complex problems like phobias, but we may be able to use some of the techniques in smaller ways.

So, for example, we might find that our patients keep reacting negatively in certain situations, such as suffering bouts of anxiety at the supermarket, or getting terrible urges to smoke every time they meet friends in a bar. By asking patients to keep a diary of *exactly* what they were doing in the moments leading up to the response, we can help them begin to find patterns and unrecognised anchors. Once anchors are recognised, patients can learn to use them to trigger different, healthier responses. This can be done initially in the imagination, and then the patient can try it in practice. NLP practitioners often get patients to anchor these preferred responses even more firmly by using ritual actions like tapping on the wrist or making eye movements.

Activity 6.2: Hypnosis in practice (1–2 hours)

For the next few patients that you see, try one or more of the following techniques.

- Preparation: actively try to calm your patients early in the consultation by creating a peaceful environment or using peaceful verbal or non-verbal language.

- Induction: use some deletions in your speech, tell short stories or use touch or body movements in unexpected ways to induce brief trance states. You can tell when these trance states happen as your patient will 'go inside' themselves temporarily.

- Intervention: use some suggestions, process instructions or hidden commands while the patient is in a trance state.

- Anchoring: work with patients to identify exactly what might be acting as negative anchors, or triggers, for their unhealthy behaviours. Try using positive suggestions and embedded commands to help them set new anchors for more healthy ones.

INTEGRATING HYPNOSIS IN PRACTICE

Our co-creations are created moment by moment. It is important to get perspective when using techniques such as hypnosis, which aim to influence patients at those moments when they are most vulnerable. While it is rare to be able to influence patients against their will, we may be able to influence patients who are ambivalent or unsure. This is a risky business when we are co-creating, because it means that one co-creator (the practitioner) has more power over the co-creation than the other co-creator (the patient).

Right values and right motivation are therefore important. We may wish to ask ourselves: am I fully aware of the patient's wishes? Am I mindful of my own motivations? Are these skilful or unskilful?

To answer some of these questions, we can try to develop and maintain a trusting rapport with our patients, so that they are able to give, and maintain, consent to the process. Without that trust and rapport, these techniques become both harder to carry out and more uncertain in their eventual effectiveness.

However, in the same way as we anaesthetise patients who are undergoing surgery, trying to enable our patients to be as calm, relaxed and open as possible when dealing with painful, traumatic or frightening areas of their life is a skilful practice, and one that is worth learning and using.

After all, when we are tired and unwell, sleep is restorative, and dreams can transform.

After Apple Picking

My long two-pointed ladder's sticking through a tree
Toward heaven still,
And there's a barrel that I didn't fill
Beside it, and there may be two or three
Apples I didn't pick upon some bough.
But I am done with apple-picking now.
Essence of winter sleep is on the night,
The scent of apples: I am drowsing off.
I cannot rub the strangeness from my sight
I got from looking through a pane of glass
I skimmed this morning from the drinking trough
And held against the world of hoary grass.
It melted, and I let it fall and break.
But I was well
Upon my way to sleep before it fell,
And I could tell
What form my dreaming was about to take.
Magnified apples appear and disappear,
Stem end and blossom end,
And every fleck of russet showing clear.
My instep arch not only keeps the ache,
It keeps the pressure of a ladder-round.
I feel the ladder sway as the boughs bend.

And I keep hearing from the cellar bin
The rumbling sound
Of load on load of apples coming in.
For I have had too much
Of apple-picking: I am overtired
Of the great harvest I myself desired.
There were ten thousand thousand fruit to touch,
Cherish in hand, lift down, and not let fall.
For all

That struck the earth,

No matter if not bruised or spiked with stubble,

Went surely to the cider-apple heap

As of no worth.

One can see what will trouble

This sleep of mine, whatever sleep it is.

Were he not gone,

The woodchuck could say whether it's like his

Long sleep, as I describe its coming on,

Or just some human sleep.

– Robert Frost[38]

Chapter 7
Dancing

Activity 7.1: People watching (1 hour)

Here's a nice one. Make some 'me-time' and go to one of your favourite haunts: maybe a café, or a pub, or a park. Order something nice, sit back and watch people go by. See what they are wearing, the gestures they use, the way they move and the space they keep around themselves. Can you see any patterns? What are they?

Now look in a mental mirror. How are you using your body?

When we are with other people we are always dancing. We co-create using our bodies just as much as our minds.

We can dance in a number of different ways,[39] for example using our facial expressions, eye movements, gestures, posture, the use of our personal space, touch or our appearance. We can also dance with our voices to give our words more meaning (by varying their speed, pitch, tone and volume).

We use our whole bodies to communicate and co-create the whole time. Our dance is both conscious but also subconscious. Being aware of our dances, and trying to understand their meanings, is a way for us to get vivid insights into each other's conscious and subconscious interior worlds, and use those insights to co-create healthier existences.

THE EFFECTIVENESS OF DANCING

Being good at dancing is also, as it turns out, a very effective and efficient skill for practitioners. If we can use and read 'body language' effectively it appears to help our patients get better quicker, be more satisfied with the outcome, miss fewer appointments, get diagnosed more quickly and accurately, stick more closely to agreed treatment plans, be more likely to get better, and less likely to sue us.[40] On the other hand, bad dancing can reduce the quality of care we provide.[41]

CULTURAL, CONTEXTUAL AND AGE DIFFERENCES

Different non-verbal signals may mean different things to different people of different ages in different places, so reading body language is not an exact science (or art). There are some expressions that seem fairly universal, such as anger, pleasure and sadness. Others, such as fear, respect, aggression or disgust are much more variably expressed.

For example, a headscarf worn by a teenage, European, male skateboarder has a different meaning compared to one worn by a middle-aged, Saudi-Arabian woman.[42] Eye contact for some may be seen as a sign of openness and trustworthiness, but for others it may be a sign of disrespect or aggression. Touch may be appropriate or inappropriate. Leaning back may be seen as a sign of comfortable friendship, or of disrespect.

> When we first went to Uganda, we were slightly taken aback by the fact that people would continuously raise their eyebrows and purse their lips at us. In the UK, eyebrow raising is sometimes a sign of surprise, or humour. Lip-pursing is often seen as a sign of hostility or even aggression. It took us a while to realise that, in Uganda, it could also mean 'I agree', or 'I understand'.[43]

As it is impossible to know exactly what anyone's non-verbal communication means, particularly if they are from a different culture or subculture, it makes sense to check back what we think they mean, for example: *'I sense that you're not quite happy with how things are progressing, is that right?'*

Of course the process is also two-way. It can be a very worthwhile exercise to ask colleagues or friends (or even friendly patients) from different cultural groups to look at us and give honest feedback about what messages we are giving off.

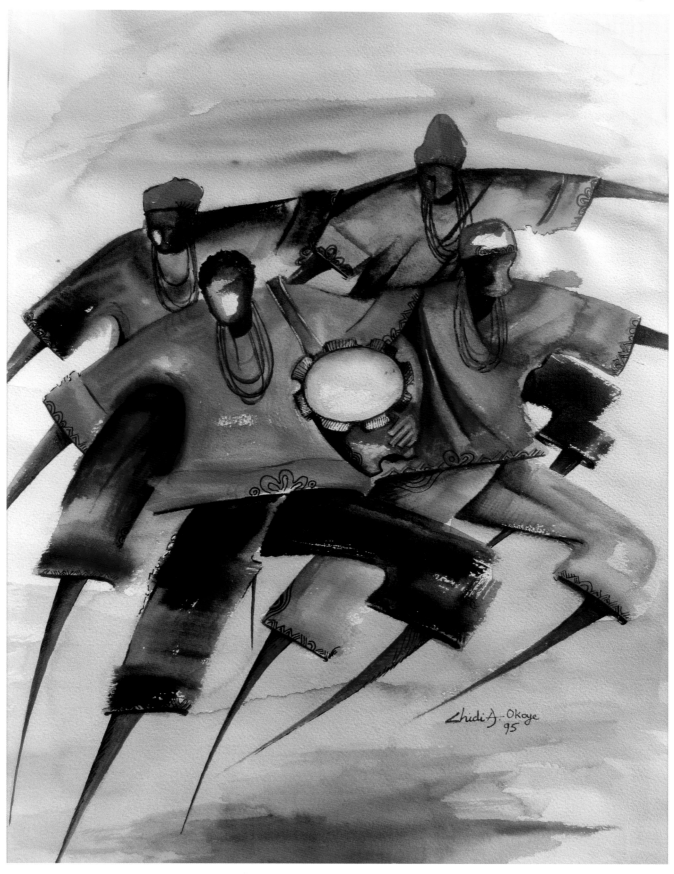

'Wind of drums' – by Chidi Okoye[44]

CUEING

If someone is not quite taking proper notice of our dancing, we can give them a poke. We might literally poke them, but most of our patients are a bit too polite for that. So they tend to poke us a bit more subtly (so subtly that sometimes they do it without realising it themselves). We call these pokes 'cues'.[45]

Cues aid our communication by poking others into closer attention, but also by adding emphasis, depth, texture and colour to our verbal messages. They can also undermine or even contradict our verbal messages, by showing an underlying ambivalence, anxiety, denial or even deceit.

Some common examples of cues that we may see in practice include a clenched fist or a chopping hand to emphasise the verbal message; body postures that either reinforce or contradict the verbal message; holding up a hand to obtain a pause; or repeating certain phrases or words to demonstrate underlying concerns.[46]

We may perform an even more subtle dance by using what are known as minimal cues.[47] These are the subtle and unconscious manifestations of our internal confusion, emotion, turbulence or dissonance. They might include[48] eye movements (particularly laterally), momentary 'trances', changes in the flow and turbulence of our voices, speech 'censoring', or the use of 'generalisations' and 'deletions' in our speech.

Some common examples of these in practice are as follows.

- Eye movements: we tend to move our eyes as we perform different functions with our brains. Try it by sitting in front of a mirror, or video yourself. Try to remember something, then do some mental maths, then think about a sad time for you, then imagine being somewhere wonderful. See how your eyes shift around.

- Trances are common in practice: and occur when patients feel some dissonance, for example due to strong emotion, or confusion (see Chapter 6 'Hypnotising' for more detail).

- Changes in flow and turbulence of our speech happen if we are distressed, angry, frightened or excited.

- Deletions are words clearly left out by the speaker, often suggesting the patient is hiding something either from themselves or from us: e.g. 'It crossed my mind that . . . but, anyway, I was hoping you could help.'

- Generalisations are phrases which are too broad or sweeping to be literally true, and which suggest possible irrational or overvalued ideation: e.g. 'I always mess up' or 'I never recover very well'.

- Value-laden phrases, which are phrases within which are embedded judgemental adjectives or nouns, and which give us a glimpse of the internal 'narratives' and 'dramas' of our patients lives: e.g. 'He's a terrible worrier' or 'She's always the strong one'.

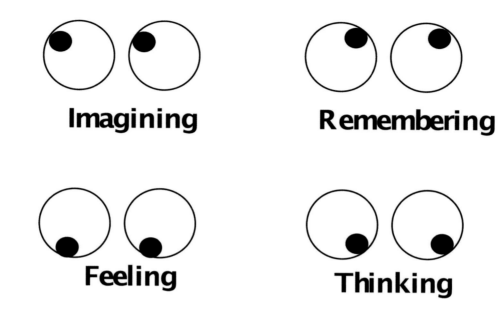

Imagining   **Remembering**

Feeling   **Thinking**

This picture demonstrates how eye movements may vary depending in the brain's activity. It is not a science, however. The movements represented here frequently occur in right-hand dominant people, but not always.

Activity 7.2: Cues (1 hour)

Picking up cues is one of the most useful, and hardest, of all consulting skills. Cues are the bridge across the gap (sometimes chasm) between our agendas and our patients' agendas. They are hard to pick up because we so easily absorbed and distracted by our own agendas and our own objectives, so we easily become blind to other possible avenues.

If you can record your consultations, try to do so. If not, try to keep a 'mental video camera' running as you consult.

As you consult, consciously look for any verbal or non-verbal cues that your patient gives you. Just for this exercise, let go of your agenda for a while and respond to them. Try to put worries about time to the back of your mind, and trust that the patient will come back to the 'right' place, albeit in their own way.

When you see or hear a cue, verbally or non-verbally show the patient that you have picked it up, and invite them to open up further. You may be amazed how much more effective, and efficient, your consultations will be.

READING BODY LANGUAGE

Reading body language is not an exact science. Body language is culturally and contextually determined, and varies from person to person. It is therefore risky to try to interpret it without checking. Part of the skill with body language lies in recognising it, but the second, equally important skill is being able to interpret and to check our interpretation with the patient. This is easily done by describing or copying back, in a questioning but non-judgemental way, what we have just witnessed.

So, for example:

- Repeating the patient's repetition: either as a sentence 'You say you are worried?' or even just the word 'worried?'
- Pointing out a deletion: 'I noticed you paused halfway through describing x. Was there something you wanted to tell me?'
- Describing back a non-verbal cue: 'I notice you chopped your hand when you were saying xx. Why was that?'

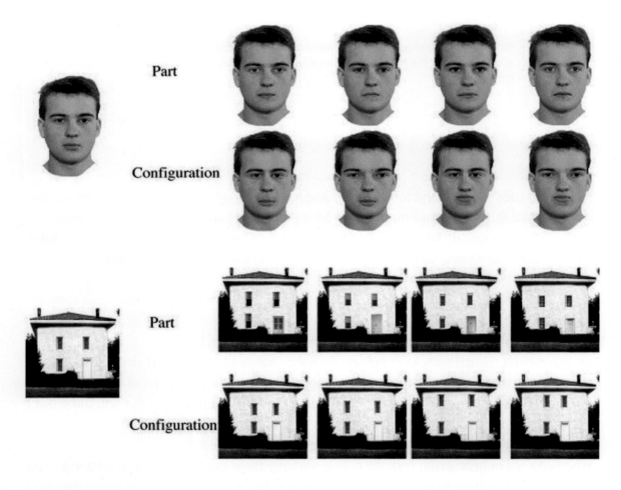

We pick up changes in facial expressions much more quickly and easily than changes in other familiar objects (such as houses in this experiment[49]). Both the faces and houses above have had parts rearranged or changed. It is much harder to pick up the differences in the houses.

- Testing out an interpretation: 'You seem quite agitated. Is that because you are finding xx upsetting, or frightening?'
- Undoing a self-contradiction: 'You said, "It's probably nothing", but what was the "something" that it possibly might be.'

SOME TIPS FOR USING OUR OWN BODY LANGUAGE IN PRACTICE

- Leaning back and putting our hands behind our head may be a sign of comfort and relaxation to us, but it may also appear as a sign of dominance.
- Finger pointing is pretty much always offensive.
- If we find our voices rising in tone or volume, cracking or becoming erratic, it's a sign to both our patients and ourselves that we need to ease up.
- Banging hands down on the table, or leaning forward with hands pressed down suggests that, if we haven't already lost it, we are just about to.
- Touch is a tricky one. A little is probably OK (as long as you're not using your fist and it's on an appropriate part of the body), but it's very personal. Some patients find it comforting, some find it off-putting and some may find it aggressive, patronising or dominant.
- A tapping, twitchy practitioner does not inspire calm or confidence.
- If you spread your arms out very wide, you are either extremely relaxed or suffering from a bad case of Messiah complex.
- If you find yourself standing with legs apart and your hands on your hips, and if you are not the patient's mother, class teacher or a police officer, you need to revisit your role definition.
- If you find yourself in an arm and leg crossing mirroring bout with your patient, you're not going anywhere, and he may be off to the lawyer.
- Eye contact is great, as long as the patient is leaning back and pupils are dilated. If he or she is leaning forward, the eye contact is intense and the eyebrows are knitted, prepare to duck.
- Matching postures is generally a good move, as long as the patient is not of the opposite sex and generally attractive to you. If he/she is, now's the time to draw the consultation to a close.
- A little head nodding and smiling is great. Too much may make you look like a buffoon!

INTEGRATING DANCE INTO OUR PRACTICE

When we dance with our patients, we co-create visual, auditory and sensory existences together. This is an incredibly valuable co-creation, which can speed us up and make us more effective in practice. The phrase 'a picture is worth a thousand words' is very apt here. A very 'thin slice' of non-verbal communication can give us insight in a fraction of a second, far more quickly and effectively than we could hope for through verbal communication alone.[50]

We therefore might find it helpful to practise our interpretation of the body language of others, but also watching and reflecting on the body language we ourselves use in practice. We can all learn to improve these skills,[51] and there are now lots of ways to do so.[52]

To make best use of body language and dancing, we need to be mindfully aware. This means being mindfully aware of the situation, avoiding coming to the consultation feeling distracted or emotional, and trying to spend as much time watching the patient as possible (rather than the screen, chart or the machine). It means being mindfully aware of ourselves, trying to dance in a way that puts patients at ease and in rapport.

Finally, it means becoming aware of what our appearances, our clothing and our environment are saying to our patients, and whether all these are integrated and balanced with the message we are trying to convey.[53]

Once we are aware of all this, we are free to begin to express ourselves through dancing with our patients and through our dance to begin to see and hear the music of our co-creation through the eyes and the ears of each other. Once we can see and hear like this, it is a small step to finding ways to dance, and to help our patients to dance, in ways that are more creative, more expressive and more healthy.

Helix

From eye unto eye
A spark.
From mind unto mind,
A dance.
From soul unto soul
A song.
From love unto love
A love.
From depth unto depth
Two strands,
Coiled
As one.

– JA

Chapter 8
Transferring and counter-transferring

Activity 8.1: Transference (30 minutes)

Find somewhere peaceful and relax. Allow your mind to clear and any emotion to settle and then clear away completely. Have a look through some pictures of faces, in a magazine, or on TV. As you look at them, become aware of the feelings that arise and disperse in you. Become aware of the possibility that these new feelings may not be your own, as your emotions were clear when you started looking at the faces. So where do they come from?

Now have a look in the mirror, and see what emotions arise now.

Some people have the ability to lift our spirits simply by entering the room, whereas others can make us instantly tetchy, euphoric, silly, bored or anxious. In the process of co-creating our existences, we seem to have the ability to 'transfer' our emotions onto other people almost instantly, often before we have even spoken. It can work two ways round.

> For example, if I feel angry inside, I might believe it is you who are angry when we meet. This is called 'transference'. You on the other hand, may feel absolutely fine until I walk in, when all of a sudden you feel inexplicably angry. That is because you are feeling my anger as if it is your own. This is called counter-transference.[54]

Transference and counter-transference are not magic. They probably happen because, when two humans meet, they unconsciously rearrange their faces and bodies to mirror the other.[55] We often think that emotions cause behaviours (like facial expressions) but, fascinatingly, it can work both ways round. Our facial expressions can also create our emotions.

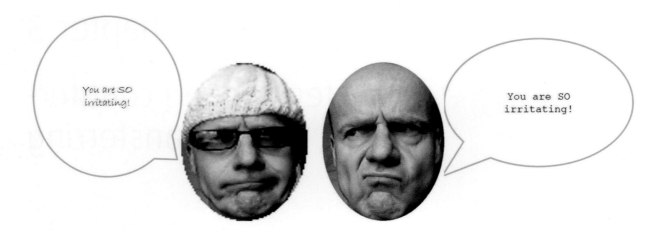

Transference and counter-transference at work

> I used to look after a lovely man, in his eighties, who was incredibly calm and gentle. This chap was a 'heart-lift' patient. The problem was he was so calming and so gentle that I would gradually go into a kind of trance when he was with me, and I would keep having to ask him to repeat what he had just said. Sadly, he died fairly recently, but even now the thought of him makes me feel peaceful.

COUNTER-TRANSFERENCE AS A TOOL

Counter-transference is arguably one of the most powerful diagnostic and therapeutic tools that we have. This is for two reasons.

First, it gives us a direct and immediate insight into what it is like to be the patient, and that is the prime aim of all health assessment. If we can think what our patient is thinking, feel what our patient is feeling, and be aware how life looks and is from their perspective, and all within the first few seconds of meeting them, we are both effective and incredibly efficient.

Second, because counter-transference is two-way, it also gives us a chance to 'reverse engineer' the patient's feelings. If we can be calm, positive and gently curious, we can help our patients feel the same. This is a very useful starting point for our therapeutic co-creation.

> A common example in practice is when we meet our 'heart-sink' patients. We can be having a great morning until the next patient comes in, and then our heart 'sinks'. We begin to feel angry, or depressed, or hopeless, for no

apparent reason. I have a particular patient who is an elderly lady for whom 'nothing works'. She seeks my help very frequently, but nothing I say or do is in any way helpful. To her everything is hopeless, and she makes me feel hopeless too! It took me a long time to realise the hopelessness belongs with her, so now I try to consciously rev myself up before and during the consultations. I do continue to try to address her hopelessness with her, but my efforts continue to be relentlessly hopeless. She still makes me feel pretty useless, but at least I can now manage to separate myself from her feelings and so allow my own feelings of empathy and sympathy to take the place of frustration and anger she used to generate in me.

Activity 8.2: 'Heart-sink' patients (30 minutes)

Relax and allow your mind and emotions to settle. When you feel calm and peaceful, bring to mind your most 'heart-sink' patient, the one who, immediately on entering the room, makes your spirit sink and your will to live expire.

Visualise every detail of his/her face, body and demeanour.

Become aware of the emotions that may be arising, or even erupting. Turn your attention away from the patient towards yourself. Remind yourself that these emotions were not there until you visualised the patient. So whose emotions are they?

Just briefly, allow yourself to see the world through that patient's eyes. How would it be to be always feeling those feelings and arousing those emotions in everyone you meet?

Then come back to yourself and move on. Be practical. Who has control?

How will you manage him or her next time you meet?

Dementor

No better doc
she says
again

No good doc
I think
again

My hope seeping,
her soul creeping
up on me

Darkness calls to darkness

In reply
my eye
sees
my light, lit

— JA

INTEGRATING TRANSFERENCE AND COUNTER-TRANSFERENCE IN PRACTICE

Transference and counter-transference, perhaps more than any other phenomenon in practice, emphasises the absolute relationality of our existence and the permeability of the boundaries of our 'selves'. Our co-creating happens without us even realising it is happening.

We cannot escape this relationality, this hidden co-creating. But we do have a choice as to whether we use our relationality as a tool or view it as a tyrant. The perspective we take is up to us. However, if we can value it, and see it as a useful tool, we can reap the reward through more effective and efficient insight into our patients and ourselves.

Our relationality, permeability and transparency can be quite troubling concepts, as they can leave us feeling vulnerable and naked. While we may be ready to deal with our patients' problems within our practice, we may be less ready to deal with our own, let alone see them reflected back at us by our patients.

Furthermore, we are not clean slates. We have our own unconscious drives, emotions and neuroses, which we can project onto the patient. This is our transference onto them. That means that if a particular emotion arises during a consultation, anger for instance, it can be very difficult to know who it belongs to. If we don't know that it is not arising from us, we can't use it. For this reason, dealing with transference and counter-transference requires a great deal of self-awareness and insight.

Transference enables us to co-create a new existence with our patients (and other people) in which our emotions are so subtly and effectively communicated we can be left unsure of what belongs with who; which can be confusing at best, and unhealthy if we find ourselves beginning to take on our patients suffering as our own.

However, if we can gain enough insight into what belongs with us, and what belongs with the patient, we can use counter-transference as an extremely useful diagnostic and therapeutic tool.

At our initial connection with patients, negative emotions may arise. However, as the connection and creation goes on, we can choose whether to respond or not to respond to those negative 'arisings', and whether to bring to consciousness new 'arisings', which are more healthy and more effective, thereby moulding our patients' (and our own) health accordingly.

Angry Man

Pulsing, pulsing
he pulses
pushing
me down, down
Shouting, shouting
he shouts
shouting
me down, down
Shrinking, shrinking
I shrink
shrinking
me down, down
Deeply, gently
we touch,
turning
us round, round

– JA

Chapter 9
Acting

Activity 9.1: Dramas in practice (30 minutes)

Think back to a dramatic consultation, one where strong emotion was generated or where your emotions came to the surface. Reflect on what happened.

It is quite possible that this won't be clear. It may even be that emotion revisits you as you remember the consultation.

But allow yourself to relax and your emotions to flow away. Rather than focus on them, consider how you were acting in that consultation. Did your actions contribute to the drama? If so, how?

Do you find you act in similar ways in other consultations? Is there a pattern?

Our co-created existences can be seen as personal, real-life 'dramas' in which we each act out our various personal roles.

Drama, like narrative, is a form of communication which seems very basic and universal in humans. Like stories, the dramas that we act out within our cultures, families and other relationships help form and support our sense of who we are.[56]

We start to dramatise and act out our ideas as small children, for whom make-believe play is a crucial form of learning, experimentation and development. As we grow up, we continue to act out dramas, although we become less aware of them.

All the world's a stage,
And all the men and women merely players:
They have their exits and their entrances;
And one man in his time plays many parts

— *As You Like It* (Shakespeare)

DRAMA IN PRACTICE

There are a number of specialist ways in which drama can be applied and used in health practice,[57] but these require more training and time than most of us have. However, a 'transactional' approach may be helpful to practitioners of all backgrounds, and at all times.

Transactional analysis suggests that there are particular cultural and familial dramas that tend to recur across society, and that are so deep rooted that we become unaware of them after early childhood. Even after we lose awareness of the script, we continue to remain subconsciously within the same 'dramas'.[58]

> If these dramas are unhealthy, it means that we can get locked in to a 'Groundhog Day' type scenario, within which we endlessly act out, with others, recurring dramas which are unhealthy for ourselves and each other. This is probably familiar for most of us. We all are aware of situations where we know we are going to act in a certain way, even before they occur. For example, there are some patients that make us feel angry, or frustrated, or demoralised, or (on the other hand) peaceful, happy or even euphoric.

As we play out our roles, either at home or at work, information flows between us and our fellow 'actors' in a conscious spoken way, but also in an unconscious and unspoken way. Berne called these flows 'transactions'. We carry out these transactions because we are subtly rewarded when we do so, for example by getting attention or by generating sensations or emotions we want. These rewards he called being 'stroked'. Strokes may be warm or cold. We prefer warm stokes (which make us feel good) but are prepared to accept cold strokes (which make us feel bad), if the only alternative is no strokes at all, because isolation is the worst of all words in the context of drama.

COMMON DRAMAS IN PRACTICE

There are many, many different dramas, but some will be particularly familiar to health practitioners.

These include, for example:

- The patient as Parent/Adult/Child
  - Parent: 'I want you to give me some tablets.'
  - Adult: 'I'd like to discuss with you what the best options are.'
  - Child: 'Oh I don't know doctor, you know best . . .'
- The Victim/Persecutor/Rescuer
  - Victim: 'Poor me doctor, no one can ever help, but I think you are different!'
  - Rescuer: 'Well, Miss Jones, that's very kind of you, and I will certainly do what I can to help.'
  - Persecutor: 'Doctor, I had such trust in you, but you've let me down like all the others; you're no better than anyone!'
  - Alternative persecutor: 'Miss Jones, I've had just about enough of you. I'm afraid there is absolutely nothing wrong with you at all, and you are just wasting my time!'
- Yes but, no but:
  - 'Yes nurse, you are quite right, that would normally work, but it didn't help with me. Thanks nurse, that's a good idea, but I'm pretty sure that won't work either. Well, nurse, you are quite right, I should exercise more, but I'm afraid my joints are just too painful.

All three of these dramas are very common in health practice. That is because they are at the heart of the problems faced by many of our patients who have what has become known as 'personality disorders' but as it is such a terrible term I'd prefer to use 'relationship difficulties' if that's OK.[59] This group of people tend to make up a very large proportion of patients attending family practice or mental health departments.[60] Furthermore, they are often what we sometimes term our 'heart-sink' patients.

People with relationship difficulties are often caught in one or more of the triangles suggested above. For example, people with dependent disorders tend to the child or victim role (and also the help-rejecting help-seeker), people with sociopathic disorders tend to the persecutor role, and people with narcissistic disorders tend to the rescuer or parent role. It is interesting to note that the health practitioner role lends itself to both the rescuer and parent roles.

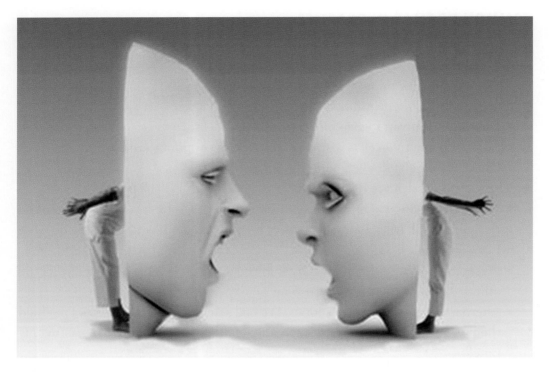

Psychodrama[61]

DRAMATIC ROLES THAT PRACTITIONERS MIGHT PLAY

As practitioners we are human beings, so we also play roles which we may or may not be aware of. Indeed we may well choose health practice as a career as it enables us to play 'parent' or 'rescuer' roles (and get plenty of 'stroking' for so doing). As health practitioners we will also often see patients who are acting out roles within dramas that are not harmonious or balanced. These roles are known as 'maladaptive roles'.

This is not a problem unless we take roles, consciously or unconsciously, that reinforce our patient's maladaptive roles.[62] We cannot step away from drama and take on a position of neutral observer, because all human interaction is a form of drama. As soon as we interact with another person, even our patients, we immediately enter another drama with them. All we can do is to become aware of our own dramas and roles, and so become aware of how our own dramas can be used to help (or harm) our patients.

When one actor in a drama comes under pressure from another actor to come out of any particular drama (for example, because they won't play their roles, or start to question them), the actors often use their psychological defences to stay within the drama. Someone playing 'victim' to another's 'persecutor' may reinterpret the persecutor's apparently kind action as manipulative abuse by an actor in the victim mode, or maybe discount it so that it does not challenge their view of themselves as victim and their co-actor as persecutor. Such 'discounting' may take the form of ignoring, becoming passive, becoming angry, becoming unsettled or agitated or even violent.

DRAMAS AS TOOL AND AS TYRANT

Because drama happens at a subconscious level, and because we do it spontaneously and naturally, drama may be a useful tool. But it can also be a dangerous tyrant. Which it is depends on our level of awareness.

If we are not aware of the drama, we may take up a role which is not healthy, and may even be harmful for the patient. Becoming aware is not at all easy, as we have built up strong psychological defence mechanisms which prevent us digging into what may lie behind the dramas we act out.[63] It is even harder if our patients act out the reciprocal roles to our own preferred role in our own drama (e.g. victim to our rescuer; or child to our parent), and have similar defences or maladaptive childhood experiences to our own.

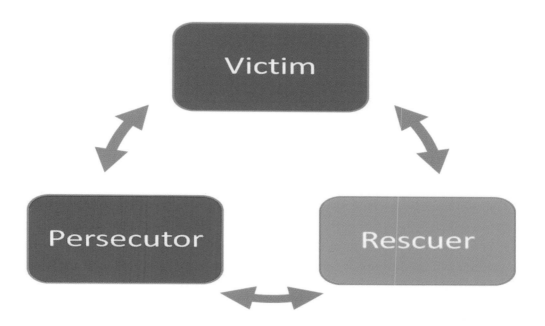

Actors often start in a favoured role, but don't necessarily stay in it. They may start in one position and switch at any moment, triggering the other actors to switch too. The result can be we get locked into a crazy game of musical chairs where the chairs never reduce, so we just go round and round the triangle. The only way out is to recognise what is going on, and refuse to play.

For example, let us take a patient who presents with one of the 'chronic pain' syndromes where no 'organic cause' has been found. It can be easy in this situation for us as practitioners to take on a range of roles, which only tend to cement the unhealthy drama. When the patient first comes with her chronic pain that no one has been able to treat, we may initially feel drawn to the rescuer role, feeling that we can succeed where others have failed, and then embarking on heroic courses of investigation or treatment. Our patient may well be happy to take the victim role overtly but she may also take on a hidden role as persecutor, punishing the practitioner (who is now victim) by ensuring all our offerings fail. As our treatment offerings fail, and as our patient steadfastly refuses to get better, we may start to get cross with our patient, either overtly (by showing our frustration) or covertly (by blocking her access to us) thereby slipping into the persecutor role. At this point the patient may retaliate by coming back, yet again, to remind us of our own inadequacy. This triangle has no end, unless we can become aware of it, and our own part in it.

On the other hand, we can turn psychodrama into a tool, by helping our patients become aware of what is going on, externalising the drama so it can be discussed and analysed in a safe way, and then using that discussion to help our patients think of different dramas that are healthier. Let's have a look at how.

INTEGRATING DRAMA INTO OUR PRACTICE

Drama can be a very useful tool for us to use as we go about the task of co-creating healthier states of existence with our patients. If we are to integrate drama in our practice, first we need to zoom out and take a detached perspective. In this regard, drama is very much like narrative, but not the same. Like narrative, we are looking to identify and externalise the story/drama. Unlike narrative, we are not taking on the role of detached 'investigative reporter'. In drama, we are an actual actor in the drama, very much part and parcel of the plot.

Therefore, to gain perspective, we can try to become 'meta-aware' of the whole drama in which we are actors. Being 'meta-aware' means being able to step off the stage and look dispassionately at the drama, like the director of a play. Once we can see the drama from the outside, including our part in it, we can begin to identify more dispassionately the plot and characters, and where the unhelpful relationships may lie. As directors rather than actors we have a much better chance of influencing the plot towards a happier and healthier ending, both for our patients and for ourselves.

For example: 'Ah, looks like I am playing rescuer to Sarah, and looks like she is persecuting me by not getting better, so I have flipped into the victim role, which has made me cross, so now I'm punishing her for not getting better, and she's back in the victim role again, but with me now as persecutor not rescuer. This is a role conflict which I don't like, as I prefer to think of myself as carer rather than bully. However, I suppose I can't ignore the evidence that I am capable of be a "bully" just as much as I am capable of being a "carer".'

Activity 9.2: Stepping off the stage (quite a long time and a lot of practice)

Go back to the consultation, or series of consultations, that you considered in Activity 9.1. This time we are going to think ahead, to the next time you feel a drama coming on.

Prepare yourself by working your way mentally through the following steps:

- **Which common role are you getting drawn into?** *(e.g. 'Hmm, I seem to always get into this rescuer position, and my surgery seems to be filling up with dependent people with intractable pain.')*

- **Consider what dynamics, concerns, worries or memories might be powering the drama? Is there anything you can do to disempower them?** *(e.g. 'Right, I wonder what I'm repressing, and what she's repressing? An abusive childhood perhaps, maybe rape, maybe sexual difficulties, maybe the upcoming wedding . . .')*

- **Try to bring the drama out into the open:** *(e.g. 'Sarah, I can't help noticing that we keep getting into similar situations, which seems to result in you getting upset and me feeling frustrated. I wonder if we should step back for a second and think about what's going on.')*

- **To look for areas of agreement and disagreement about the process, ignoring the content of the drama itself:** *(e.g. 'OK, so we agree that I tend to take to the rescuer role, and you to the victim, but both of us can make pretty good persecutors too!')*

- **Look for areas of agreement and disagreement about the process, ignoring the content of the drama itself:** *(e.g. 'OK, so we agree that I tend to take to the rescuer role, and you to the victim role.')*

- **How might you be able to negotiate your way with the patient off the stage:** *(e.g. 'Do you think it might be worth considering what else our subconscious may be hiding?')*

Play around with the ideas and actual words and body language you will use. Make sure you feel comfortable with them. Practise your lines a few times. Then step back onto the stage and try it for real.

Using drama to co-create better health is no easy task, as it requires that we value the search for truth above our own comfort and security. We have to become mindfully aware of the whole drama, including how our own psychology (and possibly psycho-pathology) is influencing the events. If we are to commit to unravelling the dramas in which we find ourselves as actors, it means unravelling not just the internal dynamics of our patient. It means unravelling our own internal dynamics as well, some of which we may be defended against for a reason.

It also requires some courage, because becoming aware of the drama is only half of the solution. We then have to come out of role and communicate, both with our patients and ourselves, what is going on and how these might reflect hidden, often very painful and well-defended problems. The reaction to this can be powerful, as patients and practitioners alike are capable of becoming powerful persecutors (and powerful victims).

However, the skilful, compassionate and courageous use of drama is an incredibly useful tool, particularly for those patients who make our hearts sink, for whom it seems as if nothing will ever work, who are addicted, who are stuck in damaging relationships, or for whom life has simply got 'stuck'. Altogether, these make up a very substantial number of our patients, so anything we can do, and any tool that we can use, to make our practice more effective is highly welcome.

Borderline Personality Disorder

my thoughts are racing
too fast for me to know
what it is I'm feeling
I wish they would flow
one minute I'm happy
smiling ear to ear
and then I get angry
and people start to fear

because after anger is violence
someone always gets the brunt
and then comes the remorse
but by then I've been shunned.
why can't I control it,
the path it always takes?
If I know it's gonna happen
can't I stop for their sakes?

the answer is no I can't
I have tried to stop before
I try to think about it

but my impulse control is poor.
Most days I'm too clingy
I hate when people leave
they think that I am bipolar
but no, I have BPD.

Borderline Personality Disorder
that's what they say is wrong
Stemming from childhood abuse
but c'mon, it's been so long!!!
Shouldn't I be better,
learned to deal with it by now?
I don't want to be like this
someone show me how.
How do I stop being angry
at people who did nothing wrong?
All these intense emotions,
I wish that they were gone.
I want to be normal
forget what's been done
to get rid of these feelings
and stop wanting to run . . .

I'm a mother now damnit
but how can I raise my kids?
I'm afraid of the world
and everything I did . . .
is how I am today
going to affect who they are?
will my mental issues
leave emotional scars?

will they hate me when they get older
for crying with no reason?

or will they love me just for trying,
and understand, inside I'm bleeding?
All these questions harass me
because all I really want
is to be a good mother
a parental confidant.

I want them to trust me
feel that I am always there
I want them to know
there isn't a secret they can't share.
But how can my kids trust me,
if I can't trust myself?
I feel like I'm torturing them
because of my mental health.

are there any suggestions
on how I can improve
the anger that is always there,
my constant bad moods?
How can I be a better mom,
a better person all around?
is it even possible to get better
and plant my feet on solid ground?

— Jessica Napoli[64]

Chapter 10
Standing and withstanding

Activity 10.1: Being overwhelmed (30 minutes)

Take some time and space to relax, and to clear your mind. Choose a moment when you feel strong.

Think back to a time where you felt utterly overwhelmed in practice, where your foundations crumbled and you struggled to keep your balance.

As you remember, emotions may arise. Allow them, but don't engage, just watch them arise and subside. Take note of them.

Turn your mind to yourself. Become aware that you are still here, still standing, despite it. Have a good inner look at yourself. What is it about you that enables you to stand, and withstand, even when your practice is overwhelming?

Meditate for a while on the value of standing, and of withstanding, in practice.

I can think of many reasons not to like these books, but perhaps the greatest of these is the sense they may give that everything can be fixed: with the right trick, the right approach, or the right perspective.

In which case, let's just take a small step back and a salutary look around.

Every now and again we co-create states of existence with our patients that we are not prepared for, nor aware of, and over which we have absolutely no control. Being completely out of control is frightening for anyone, particularly for health practitioners like us, as we tend to like to feel in control.

Uncontrolled and uncontrollable moments can burst straight through our veneers and remind us that, whatever we do, and however well we do it, we will not be able to prevent suffering, cruelty, pain or death for many of our patients. These moments often arise without warning, can be very frightening in their power and intensity, and usually occur right in the middle of a 'typical' day.

Co-creations they may well be, but they are co-creations that can threaten to turn on us and overwhelm us.

While we can't avoid them, or control them, we can at least try to prepare ourselves by imagining them, and imagining ourselves within them. This kind of mental preparation can help us be better able to cope with terrible events when they happen, a bit like soldiers training for the horrors of war by acting out war games.

Imagination is not a rational activity, and so I am not sure that trying to engage with these issues on a rational level is helpful. But there are other, non-rational, but nevertheless valuable ways of engaging with profound pain and emotion. In this chapter, I'm not even going to attempt to offer useful evidence, theories or useful suggestions. I am simply going to use poetry as a tool, and hope that it works for you.

DEATH

Considering how common it is, especially in our line of work, death still holds a power over us. Losing a loved one rips us open, so that we can never fully heal.

Familiar

The familiar sight
Of a child dying before me
A frozen moment of infinite peace
Before reality shatters
And shards of pain
Slice open

The familiar feel
Of my own suffocation
As the witch begins her feast
From the inside
Starting with
My heart

– JA

HORROR

Sometimes, our patients may be perpetrators or victims of terrible cruelty, and with them the full horror of life can stride unannounced into our practice.

Lesley Anne
I read today
The final words of Lesley Anne

Such cruelty
Such suffering

Imagining it, one can hardly go on
But one can hardly go on, without imagining

– JA

RAGE

Our patients do not always meet pain and suffering with equanimity. Unannounced, anger can flare up. Our patients' rage may be so blind we cannot determine if it is aimed at us, or even if it arises within us.

Do not go gentle into that good night

Do not go gentle into that good night,
Old age should burn and rave at close of day;
Rage, rage against the dying of the light.

Though wise men at their end know dark is right,
Because their words had forked no lightning they
Do not go gentle into that good night.

Good men, the last wave by, crying how bright
Their frail deeds might have danced in a green bay,
Rage, rage against the dying of the light.

Wild men who caught and sang the sun in flight,
And learn, too late, they grieved it on its way,
Do not go gentle into that good night.

Grave men, near death, who see with blinding sight
Blind eyes could blaze like meteors and be gay,
Rage, rage against the dying of the light.

And you, my father, there on that sad height,
Curse, bless, me now with your fierce tears, I pray.
Do not go gentle into that good night.
Rage, rage against the dying of the light.

—Dylan Thomas[65]

SADNESS

We are usually prepared for a little emotion, although even this may make us feel uncomfortable. But sometimes we witness emotion that is so powerful, so raw, we feel as though we may be flayed bare.

Song making

My heart cried like a beaten child
Ceaselessly all night long;
I had to take my own cries
And thread them into a song.

One was a cry at black midnight
And one when the first cock crew –
My heart was like a beaten child,
But no one ever knew.

Life, you have put me in your debt
And I must serve you long –
But oh, the debt is terrible
That must be paid in song.

– Sarah Teasdale

FUTILITY

We like to be able to fix things, to find hope, to cheer up our patients. Sometimes, though, the cumulative pain and loss that we witness, and partake in, triggers such a profound sense of futility that it sucks away our optimism and threatens to dry us up.

Oh let me be alone

Oh let me be alone, far from the eyes and faces
Let me be alone, a while, even from you:
My soul is like a desert, sick of light filled spaces,
The urge of useless winds, the skies of pitiless blue:
Let me be alone, a while, in twilight places,
Waiting the merciful night, the stately stars
And the dew

— Sarah Teasdale

POWERLESSNESS

As practitioners, we have a lot of power and authority. This is helpful, both for us and our patients. But from time to time, someone lifts the corner of the curtain and we get a glimpse of forces that render us so puny and powerless that we have no choice but to surrender.

The House that Fear Built: Warsaw, 1943

The purpose of poetry is to remind us how difficult it is to remain just one person, for our house is open, there are no keys in the doors . . .

Czeslaw Milosz (*Ars Poetica*)

*I am the boy with his hands raised over his head
in Warsaw.*

*I am the soldier whose rifle is trained
on the boy with his hands raised over his head
in Warsaw.*

*I am the woman with lowered gaze
who fears the soldier whose rifle is trained
on the boy with his hands raised over his head
in Warsaw.*

*I am the man in the overcoat
who loves the woman with lowered gaze
who fears the soldier whose rifle is trained
on the boy with his hands raised over his head
in Warsaw.*

I am the stranger who photographs
the man in the overcoat
who loves the woman with lowered gaze
who fears the soldier whose rifle is trained
on the boy with his hands raised over his head
in Warsaw.

The crowd, of which I am each part, moves on
beneath my window, for I am the crone too
who shakes her sheets
over every street in the world
muttering

What's this? What's this?

— Jane Flanders[66]

LOVE

When we find ourselves in these situations, we may feel an urgent wish to 'do' or to 'say' something to 'make it better', to create peace and happiness where there is none. This is understandable, and is perhaps a sign of our love and empathy for our patients and for life.

But the problem is that, sometimes, perhaps even often, there is really nothing we can say or do to make the problem better. The creation is too strong and we are too weak. To pretend otherwise is to deny our patients their reality, and to undermine their response. At such times, all we can do is to try to stand, and to withstand, alongside our patients.

At such times, perhaps our practice is best summed up as 'skilful compassion'. We can sometimes lose sight of this, with all the other demands and frustrations of what we do. But at moments like this, when we witness and feel the terrible pain of our patients, we are prompted to remember that we do have compassion, that we do love, and that we do have a choice.

We can care, and risk suffering the pain of that caring; or we can avoid caring at all.

Without love, we cannot care, either for our patients or for each other. If at times we too rage, or feel bereft, or horrified, or powerless, or futile with our patients, at least it is a sign that we still feel love. And if we can find ways of expressing that love, in as skilful a way as possible, we can be proud of what we do, even when it is not anywhere near enough.

Caring

Softly
Beats the gentle heart
In the hardness

Quietly
Speaks the soul's small voice
In the din

Strongly
Burns our compassion
In the suffering

To fight, amour bound, but soul imprisoned?
To flee, soul free, but world divorced?

Bravely,
Beats the gentle heart
Creating softness

Honestly,
Sings the courageous soul
Creating harmony
Gently
Into suffering
With compassion

– JA

Activity 10.2: Why do you care? (30 minutes)

This might be tricky, but we have now come a long way together, so it's time to be honest and open up. Why do you care?

Forget the bravado and bluster. OK, it's a good job. It pays the bills. We quite enjoy the power and admiration. If we are honest we also have a pretty good-going Martyr or God complex going.

But deeper than that. Why do you care?

Let's meditate for a while. We are going inside.

Find a quiet place and allow your tension to drain and your breathing to settle. As you do, start to pay more attention to your breath. Feel it just inside the tip of your nose. Cold, then warm. Cold, then warm. Enjoy that for a while.

Now follow it deeper. Feel the muscles of your throat subtly shift. Backward then forward. Backward then forward. Notice the slight turbulence as the air flows past, and how that turbulence changes with the in-breath and then the out-breath. Course, then smooth. Course, then smooth. Ride with that for a while.

Follow it deeper still, to the dark depths of your diaphragm. Watch as it slowly, gently but firmly rises and falls, rises and falls. Allow that movement to pull you deeper with every in-breath and soothe you with every out-breath.

Now become aware of a depth, a presence, deep in the centre of your chest. In here is the heart of who you are. Watch it for a while and see how it gradually surges with the in-breath and eases with the out-breath.

As you watch, feel yourself getting drawn closer and closer to it, so it becomes clearer and clearer. As you get close notice how its outer shell begins to melt away, revealing more and more of the light that is inside you, of the love that is inside you, that is you.

Ignore the inner voice of cynicism. Throw off the protective shell.

If you didn't still care, if you didn't still love, you wouldn't be reading this book.

Spend some time considering that light, that love, and congratulate yourself that it is still burning, despite everything.

Chapter 11
Playing

Activity 11.1: Play (30 minutes)

Do you still play? Of course you do? How?

More importantly, do you play enough?

Think about your practice. Does it give you any opportunities for playing? If not, why not? We know what happens to boys (and girls) who don't play, don't we?

List a few things you could do to incorporate more play and fun in your work.

Co-creation can be fun. Indeed perhaps we should say co-creation *ought* to be fun. We know that all work and no play makes Jack a dull boy. Nobody wants a dull practitioner, and no-one wants to be one either.

As practitioners we work a lot, but do we play enough? The opportunity is certainly there in our practice if we want it. Most of us look after children, who are always keen to play. Most of us also look after some quite playful adults, who are usually happy to join in with a bit of tomfoolery.

> I have an admission to make. There is an elderly lady on my list who has an outrageous yet hilarious view of the world. She teases me mercilessly, and she always makes me laugh. I make sure I see her every few months, even if there is nothing wrong with her . . .

But play is not just for fun. It is seriously useful too. It can help us to make sense of the world around us, to 'practise' for 'real life', to act as a catharsis, to experiment with and get control of our hidden thoughts, to support our development, to experience a sense of freedom and control, to manipulate our reality and to feel empowered.

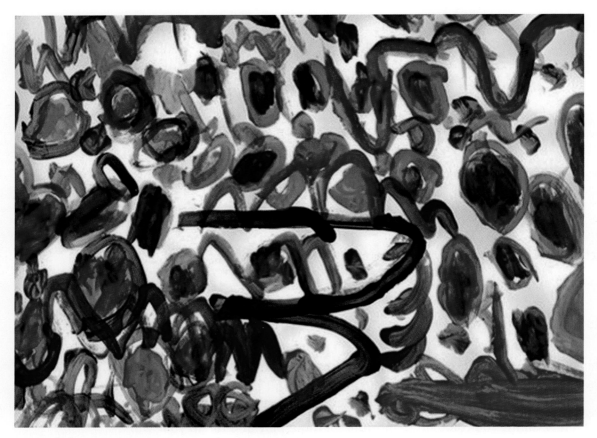

'When I am feeling cross' – by Katende Emmanuel, aged 5

CHILDREN AND PLAY

However, let's start with the experts: children.

> In some parts of the world, children make up more than half the population, yet it is rare to see anything about communication with children in communication skills materials for practitioners. This seems odd. It's almost as if they don't count as much.

As we all know, children speak three languages: verbal, non-verbal and play. It follows that, if we can't speak 'play language', we may be reducing our ability to co-create with our child patients.

There are many theories about play. It allows children to practise for later life, but there seems to be much more to it than that.[67] There are many different types of play, and each type has different positive effects[68] and encourages the development of different skills and abilities.[69]

We cannot all be play specialists, and we may not be able to devote large amounts of time to playing (*worst luck*), but at least we can try to create some time, some space and some tools to allow children (and others) to play, so that we can obtain a fascinating, and crucial, insight into their worlds.

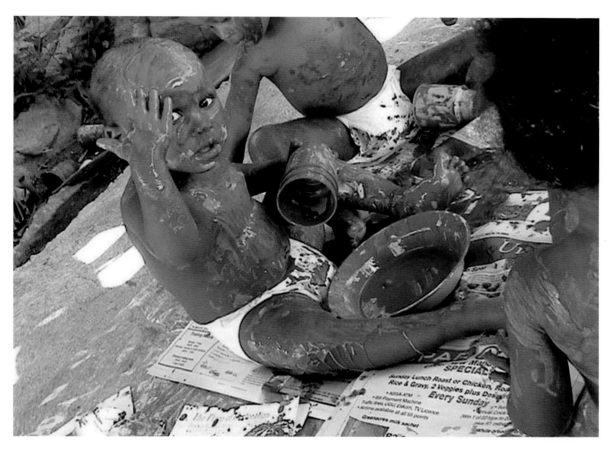

'Painting' with thanks to Sue Boucher!

PLAY AND DEVELOPMENT

Children are not simply 'mini-adults'. They see, feel and experience the world in a different way; use different thought processes to interpret it; and communicate and act differently to adults. If we don't understand this, we will find it very hard to understand children or to be understood by them.[70]

Children learn from the way they see and experience their world; from the way people treat them; and from what they see, hear and experience from the moment they are born. Children are natural learners. Between birth and five years, children grow and learn at the fastest rate of their lifetime (the so-called 'critical learning period'[71]).

Play has all the characteristics of a fine and complete educational process. No other activity motivates repetition more thoroughly. It develops initiative, imagination and intense interest. There is tremendous intellectual ferment, as well as complete emotional involvement. No other activity improves the personality so markedly. No other activity calls so fully on the resources of effort and energy which lie latent in the human being. Play is the most complete of all the educational processes for it influences the intellect, the emotions and the body of the child. It is the only activity in which the whole educational process is fully consummated, when experience induces learning and learning produces wisdom and character.[72]

THE IMPORTANCE OF PLAY IN VULNERABLE CHILDREN

Play helps children makes sense of, act out and practise new forms of existence, particularly unpleasant forms of existence, like ill health. But children who are unwell, or who are coping with difficult family or social circumstances, often miss out on play opportunities. This is a double-whammy, as they need to play even more than

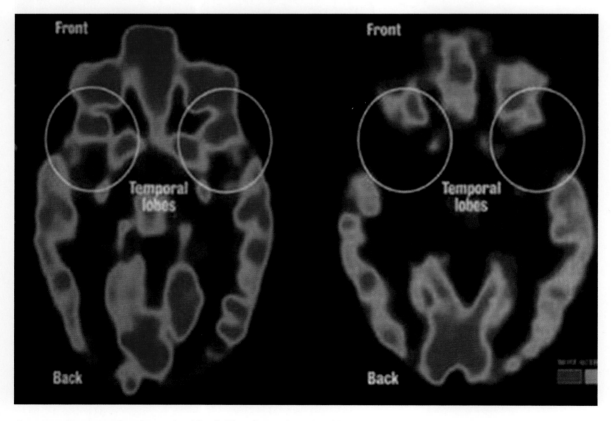

These are PET scans taken from a healthy (left) and a neglected child (right). We don't need to be specialists to see what profound impact under-stimulation can have on a child.

healthy children, in order to help them cope and come to terms with their difficult existences.

Disturbances such as long-term ill health can significantly affect the development of young children on all levels, whether physical, perceptual, cognitive, linguistic, social, emotional, moral or spiritual.[73] If these disturbances occur in early life, they can even cause permanent structural damage to the brain, and impeded future development.

REMEMBERING HOW TO PLAY

Because play is so essential, and because we are highly likely in our practice to come across children with chronic ill-health, family break-up, trauma or abuse, we have an enormous responsibility, and also a tremendous opportunity. We can make a profound difference in the life and the development of children, simply by playing and having fun. Isn't that a wonderful idea? Yet most health workers feel anxious about playing with children and lack confidence in how to go about it.

> But here's the thing. We don't need to 'know' anything. That's just sooooo 'adult'!

Play is about letting go, and doing whatever you fancy, at the time you fancy, and without caring in the slightest about who thinks what about it.

When we become adults, we tend to become more self-conscious, and more serious, and so we forget how to play. We are so used to learning and being trained, we feel anxious about playing because we don't feel 'trained' to do it.

> I remember after my first child was born. I'd kitted out the playroom, and made sure he had all the correct kind of toys, to stimulate the correct parts of his brain, at the correct stages, according to the correct books, from the correct sources. But the little bugger wouldn't play along. I'd try to set up this, and he'd want to do that. I'd pick up a book. He'd pick up a box. I'd pick up the box. He'd move on to a book. It would drive me almost mad with frustration. He just wouldn't 'get it'.

Children don't get trained to play. They are naturals at it. But they are surprisingly good, and incredibly patient, trainers. If we can just manage to throw off all the corsets and constraints of adulthood, and just sit quietly with them, they will soon teach us what to do next.

> By the time my fifth one came along, I'd given up. The best I could do was lie on the floor of the playroom (by now a wasteland of fantastically coloured plastic, half sets of puzzles, defunct electrical toys, 10,000 dead batteries,

half-chewed dried-up felt-tips, dog-eared books and enough free McDonald's toys to create an army) in the hope of catching some sleep while pretending to do my child-care shift. And that's when I finally cracked it. Of course the little tyrants were not going to let me sleep. It was 'Dad, Dad, Dad, Dad': question after suggestion after question after suggestion. Their games, their questions, their plans, their terms.

Now I have perfected the art of playing flat on my back with one eye open.

PLAYING IN PRACTICE

OK, so maybe we can't lie on the floor of our consulting rooms or wards and pretend to play while catching up on sleep. But there is nothing to stop us consulting from the floor of our consulting rooms or wards. And there is nothing to stop us having a few bits and pieces that children can play with while we talk to their parents (while watching the children – it's amazing how much clinical information you can get just by watching a child play).

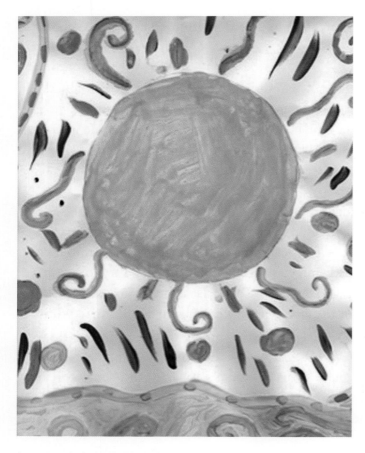

'Happiness' – by Nonnie, aged 10

The key is to ensure that children don't see us as a threat. In most cases, this is really just a question of smiling and being warm and polite with their parents or carers.

Once children can see that we are relatively safe, and that their parents are at ease with us, they almost always come to us when they are ready. They may literally come to us, or they may start to engage from the other side of the room, or their pushchair, or wherever.

If they don't come, or if they come too quickly and without checking us out first, that might be interesting in itself. Once they are engaged, all we have to do is respond to whatever they offer. If they smile, we smile. If they pull a face, we pull a face. If they wave, we wave.

They are in control of play, because they are the experts. We just respond and learn. Simple.

The most important thing we can do is to encourage, include and congratulate, encourage, include and congratulate: for saying hello, for their smart shoes, for helping Mum to explain, for showing you their foot, for allowing you to look in their ear, for helping you get the paper out of the printer, or for holding the torch when you don't need it.

USEFUL STUFF

Realistically, in the business and busy-ness of health practice, we are not going to have a huge amount of time to do much playing. So our play is going to have to be in 'thin slices'. But we can learn a lot in a mindful few moments with a child, and they can learn a lot about us. We also probably won't have a huge amount of space.[74] But we don't need much of that either. Just a very small child-friendly zone and a box with a few basic bits and pieces.

It also might help to have a few clues about what might work with different age groups. This isn't training – we can still let the children lead the way – but they are simply tips.

- From 0 to 18 months: copy their sounds; make eye contact and smile with them; allow them to play with your fingers; play 'peek-a-boo' and 'bye-bye'; look and make faces; lose, find and name things; shake a rattle or a bunch of keys; encourage them to crawl to toys out of their reach. Have a couple of picture books, rattles, stacking toys or blocks, materials of different textures, large soft toys or dolls.
- From 18 months to 3 years: give them space to move around; have them search for things in a toy box; keep a few wooden blocks, some large crayons and paper, a soft ball, or picture books so that they can play while you talk. Children this age love naming, so you can play 'name and examine' with body parts, or clothes, or toys. Copy examinations on Mum or on a toy before on them. Guessing games are great. Give them your stethoscope or torch to copy you, put them in stories about children who are sick, deliberately get names wrong and see if they correct you. Let them help you by holding or getting things.
- For 3–6 year olds: children this age have a great sense of the ridiculous. They love it if you get things wrong or make mistakes. They are getting into friends

and school, so they like to tell you about their best friends, or their teachers. They may find it easier to speak on the toy phone than to your face; or to have make-believe conversations. They can be involved in the examination by doing it themselves, holding things, looking at your watch and helping you count. They also like naming body parts and finding out what each bit does. Useful bits and pieces might include Plasticine or play-dough, crayons and paper, colours and shapes, action figures and dolls, large puzzles, toy cars and machines, simple musical instruments, blocks, buttons, and dressing up clothes.

- For 6–12 year olds: children this age still love all the funny and daft stuff, but also want to be taken a bit more seriously. They hate being patronised and are usually considerably smarter than we are. Head-patting, hair-ruffling and cheek-pinching are out. Respecting space is in. Asking them what they think, and involving them by explaining what you think, helps build trust. Get permission for everything, and respect the 'no'. Use the consultation as a teaching session about the body and health, organising and classifying things, and recounting stories about other children you have seen are all helpful. Gentle teasing often works, but for the more confident ones. They also love seeing you mess up and make mistakes, so a bit of gentle clowning is often appreciated, as are nonsense words, jokes and riddles. Books, fantasy toys, toy cars and machines, puzzles, disused phones or keyboards, sport stuff and dressing up stuff can be useful.

Activity 11.2: Playing in practice (30 minutes)

Have a little think about how you can use play more in your practice. It doesn't have to be just with children, but let's focus on children here. Think about what you can change in:

- the area you consult, to make it more child friendly
- any bits and bobs you can carry round or bring in to aid play
- any ways that you can learn more of the 'language of play'
- some specific things you might do to integrate more play into your practice
- most importantly, how you can improve your attitude and approach to children.

INTEGRATING PLAY IN PRACTICE

For many of us, our practice has become a very serious affair, and co-creating better health a rather turgid business. But it doesn't have to be like this. We can have fun as we co-create with our patients. In this regard, children have a lot to teach us.

It is natural to feel a little nervous with children, because they are vulnerable, communication is not so easy, and they may act out. But we can try to take perspective. We've all been children (*some of us longer ago than others*), and we can all remember the pure pleasure of playing. We deserve a bit of fun from time to time, so we can see child patients as an opportunity to enjoy ourselves, while getting paid for it.

In many countries of the world, children make up a very large proportion of patients. In all countries, children have disproportionately higher levels of illness, death, accident, abuse and neglect than adults. So being able to communicate with them – play with them – is something of great value that is worth some commitment and dedication.

Even better than that, it is just about the only medical skill we don't have to learn. In fact we have to un-learn. If we can be mindfully aware enough of our own inhibitions, and our own vanity, and our own anxiety, we might feel able to gingerly step out and have a go.

If we can, we might find that not only do we open up a whole new range of co-creation, we have fun doing so, and we learn from the experts – the children – who are just about the most patient and forgiving teachers we can get.

Playing

On a warm summer's day we play out with a ball,
Pretend games with toys we like best of all.
Skipping and dancing all such fun,
When you begin to play you know that you've won!
You feel so unstoppable playing with a friend,
Because you know when you play the fun will not end.

When you're feeling sick and you're spirits are low,
Playtime is out there you should know.
It will warm you're heart and be rid of your frown,
Because when you play happiness is all around!!

– Florence, aged 10

Chapter 12
Ritualising

Activity 12.1: Rituals in practice (20 minutes)

Rituals aren't just about religion. We use rituals all the time.

Have a think about your practice. You almost certainly use rituals.

What are they?

Do you ever feel that practice has become ritualistic, that we seem to be going through the same rites, over and over, without really understanding why?

Perhaps that is because it is, and we are, and we don't?

WHAT ARE RITUALS?

As we go about the business of creating and co-creating our existences, it is not surprising that we tend to lapse into habitual, almost ritualistic routines. So let's pause for a moment to consider rituals in health practice, and see if they have anything of value to teach us.

A ritual is a symbolic 'acting out' of our internal personal, familial and cultural beliefs and values.

To 'outsiders' rituals can seem meaningless or even absurd. Even to 'insiders' they may be difficult to explain.[75] In a way, they are like narratives, but at a group or cultural level. They are symbolic entities that seem to signify the shared stories and meanings of groups, linking us to each other in the present, to our ancestors in the past and to our progeny in the future.

Rituals seem particularly to be associated with times of transition, for example births, marriages, deaths, inaugurations and partings. However, they can also be associated with much more minor transitions. Examples might include the fact that most of us get dressed in exactly the same order every morning (transiting from night to day), having a 'nice cup of tea' (transiting from upset to not upset), going to the pub or to the match at the weekend (transiting from work to play), shaking hands or saying 'hello' when we meet (transiting from me to we).

Of course we don't exactly know why we use rituals in this way, but theorists have speculated that it may be because rituals offer us a comforting point of familiarity and certainty that helps us to cope with, and make sense of, changes to our existence.[76]

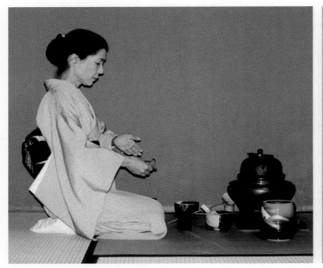 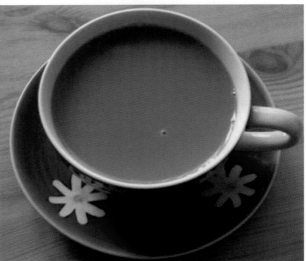

The tea ceremony in Buddhist cultures is a ceremonial ritual intended to create harmony, peace and discipline. Much of the discipline and ceremony has gone out of the British 'nice cup of tea', but the ability of British tea to create harmony and peace (especially when someone is upset, tired or otherwise down in the dumps) is still going strong!

Activity 12.2: The match your practice game (30 minutes)

Unfortunately, I can't find any evidence of the possible significance of ritual in health practice, so I am going to have to resort to anecdote.

Some time ago I took time out of practice to study theology. One of the essays I had to write was on 'ritual in my practice'. All my classmates on the course were priests or ministers of some description or other, so this was fairly simple for them. As a doctor however, I didn't feel I had much to say on the subject. In fact I felt rather hard done by and let my tutor know that. However, my tutor asked me to give it a go, and I was surprised by what I found.

To give you an idea, I have put together a matching game (*see* the table below) comparing the standard family practice consultation in the UK with the ritual of Holy Communion in the Christian church.

It's actually quite enlightening. Please have a go at matching the elements together.

(I've done the first one for you . . .)

Personal preparation	→	Personal preparation
Vicar robes up		Reassurance and advice given
Congregation arrives		Patient is dismissed
Confession		Deeper discussion of complaints
Prayers and hymns		Doctor dons white coat and prepares room and equipment
Sermon		Examination
Blessing of the sacraments		Doctor feeds data into the computer
Worshippers come to the altar		Patients booked in to surgery
Laying on of hands		The prescription is issued
Absolution		Patient presents complaint
The bread and wine		Patient gives thanks to doctor
Thanksgiving		Patient is dismissed
Dismissal		The doctor gives an opinion

INTEGRATING RITUALS INTO OUR TREATMENT

We can take different perspectives about rituals. In philosophy and theology theorists tend to take opposing view. Some, for example Freud, see them as redundant and infantile hangovers from our childhood. Others, for example Durkheim, see them as useful cultural forms of storytelling and drama that integrate us, balance us and help us deal with complexity and transition.

If we see them as the latter, we may value rituals as therapeutic in and of themselves. Becoming sick is a major transition in life, and usually a very unpleasant and unwelcome one. If the theories about rituals performing an important role in helping us through transitions are right, perhaps we can see ritual as a very useful and helpful tool in co-creating better health. After all, it seems that going to see a health practitioner is, in many ways, a ritual, and it seems clear that we health practitioners use ritualistic processes as part of our practice (although we may not realise it). Therefore we may as well look at it positively as negatively.

As practitioners, by becoming mindfully aware of the rituals we use as part of our practice, perhaps we can become more aware of how patients do (or do not) 'buy in' to our rituals. By taking this perspective, maybe we can get a better insight into their deeper view of the world, into their sense of personal and cultural identity, into their sense of belonging within our society, and into the transitions and life crises that they are currently undergoing.

By asking ourselves which rituals we currently use, and perhaps which rituals we could use, we can add another tool to our creative toolkit. Ritual may be a tool that helps our patients to find structure, purpose, belonging and meaning at a time of chaos, fear, detachment and uncertainty. In learning and practising ritual within and as part of our practice, perhaps we may be able to become more effective (and integrated) practitioners.

Ritual

Obeying the call
we congregate
to reveal
your faults
concealed
Hands laid on
we become
whole
as one
at-one
Our prescription
a benediction
we release,
healed,
in peace

— JA

Chapter 13
Motivating

Activity 13.1: Bad habits (30 minutes)

If you are like me, you will have a number of bad habits.

So why don't you just stop?

It's not so easy, is it? We get something from the bad habits, and it's not just guilt.

Have you ever tried to stop and failed? If so, spend some time considering why that might be.

Have you ever tried to stop and succeeded? If so, spend some time considering why that might be too.

In our co-creative partnership with patients, we sometimes wish to influence them in ways that we believe will make them healthier, but which they are resistant to take. At other times, patients do wish to change, but find they do not have the resources to change without help.

THE IMPORTANCE OF 'SELF EFFICACY'

There are a number of techniques that we can use to help our patients who have become 'stuck' to create healthier states of existence for themselves. Most of these techniques focus on building what has become known as the 'self-efficacy' of the patient. Self-efficacy is basically our capacity to make necessary change happen. It is a function of our strength, energy and self-belief. Self-efficacy influences our choices, the effort we may put into our choices, and how we feel about those choices before, during and after we carry them out.[77] We can build self-efficacy in many ways: from experience, by observing others, or being persuaded by those we trust.

Our experiences can create either virtuous or vicious circles. If we have positive and successful experiences of change, our self-efficacy builds, we feel better about ourselves, and we are consequently more likely to be successful next time. If we have negative experiences of change, the reverse happens, we feel worse about ourselves, and we are less confident and less willing to change the next time.

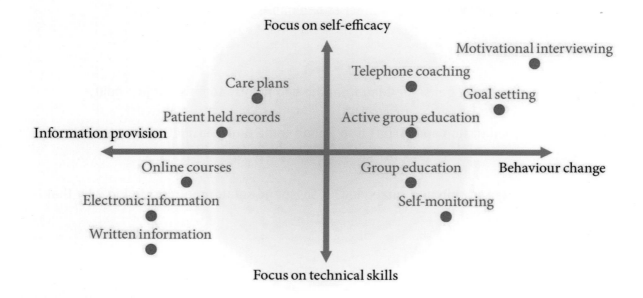

From: *Evidence: helping people help themselves. A review of the evidence considering whether it is worthwhile to support self-management* (Health Foundation, May 2011)[78]

MOTIVATING OUR PATIENTS

As practitioners we often see patients with smoking, alcohol and drug addictions, or who are trying to lose weight or get fit, or who are having difficulty taking their medications regularly, or who have problems keeping appointments.[79]

> Few of us like to be told what to do, and many of us (well, me at least) stubbornly resist change unless we decide to do it for ourselves.

Unfortunately, as discussed elsewhere in these books, the choices we make about our health are highly relational and can be influenced by numerous motivations and drives, not all of which are conscious, and many of which may be contradictory. The contradictory nature of our drives leave most of us with habits we would rather not have, and yet also a state of ambivalence about the prospect of trying to change.

As practitioners, simply telling our patients to stop doing something is not always effective (although it does make some difference[81]). If we can help our patients increase their own internal motivation, it appears we can improve on that by using another fairly directive form of communication. This is called motivational interviewing, for which increasing evidence is emerging.[82]

Motivational interviewing is based upon the idea that, when we try to change part of ourselves or our lives, it is not an 'all or nothing' event. Rather, we go through different stages.[83]

1   Not even being aware of the need to change
2   Thinking about change
3   Trying (and often failing) to change
4   Eventually succeeding (or giving up).

We can go up and down this list, and there is no guarantee that we will get all the way to success.

By accepting that we are all ambivalent, that most of us have some addictive behaviour or another, and by trying to help patients along the process of change, the whole issue can be less undermining for patients and less frustrating for us as practitioners.

If we can refrain from being judgemental (i.e. by showing that we accept our patients as they are, with the contradictions they have) we can sometimes find our relationship with our patients is strong enough for them to accept our motivation to change. In this trusting and non-judgemental relationship, we may be able to be fairly directive about trying to get the patient to recognise, examine and resolve their ambivalence, so that change becomes possible.

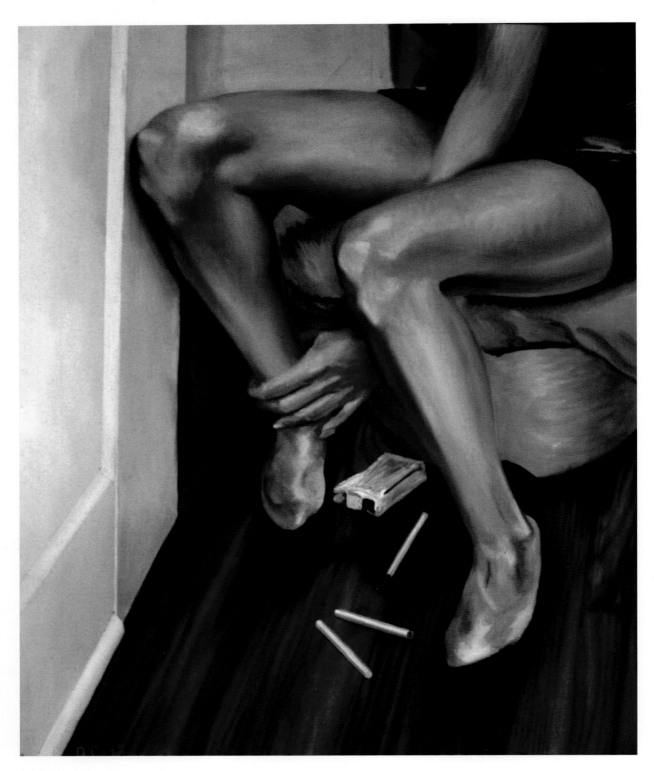

'Bad Habits' – by Dwayne Carter[80]

DISCREPANCY

The key aim of motivational interviewing seems to be to look for and then point out *discrepancies* between what the patients says they wish or hope for in their future and the likely outcomes of the direction they are currently heading.

By creating strong rapport and expressing empathy, we can build a trusting relationship with our patients that is strong enough to deal with the ups and downs of change.

> Let us take, for example, a patient of mine we can call Louise. She's a drug addict, currently holding down a job, but struggling. She is narcissistic, so not easy to like, but she also suffers with low self-esteem and also carries a lot of pain from abuse in her childhood, so it is easy to feel sympathetic towards her.
>
> She once came to see me for a repeat prescription of her oral contraceptive pill. I was doing OK for time and personal energy, so I decided to bring up the addiction. Louise, like many patients who have addictions or unhealthy lifestyles, is fed up with being lectured at and I knew from last time that she would be quite hostile to this line of enquiry. So, having recently watched a YouTube video about motivational interviewing (YouTube currently appearing to be my main source of medical training) this time I just smiled, made eye contact, relaxed back, and started with an open question: 'Anyway, here's the prescription. I've got a few minutes so it would be good to hear how you are doing in yourself?'

Once we have rapport and our patient's trust, we can begin to ask questions about what issues may motivate the change, and what issues prevent change. This is the skilful bit, as the practitioner starts to introduce ideas that support change, but without the patient feeling coerced. There are numerous 'change questions' we could ask, for example:
- 'What is the worst thing that could happen?'
- 'How was life before?'
- 'I wonder what life will be like for you after you xxx.'

During this process, we may meet resistance and failure, but we can 'roll with it' by slightly withdrawing in the face of hostility, and advancing in the face of openness, but always maintaining a non-critical and trusting relationship, based on the belief that the patient is capable of change, but that it is the patient, not the practitioner, who is responsible for that change.

> Initially hostile and aggressive, with a fair bit of swearing, Louise gradually settled down and got to the end of her story. I summarised back, partly to check, partly to show I was listening without judging: 'So, things have been

quite tough, you're in trouble at work, you've been short of money, you slept with someone to get more money, and now you are feeling partly angry, partly disgusted with yourself, and partly really, really sad?'

After a while, it might become apparent that, despite their initial defensiveness, our patients in fact do feel a lot of ambivalence towards their problem. It may be that they can see lots of reasons not to change, but they can also see reasons why change might be helpful. This is called 'discrepancy' between their actions and their desires. Discovering and exploring discrepancy is at the heart of motivational interviewing.

'I can see why you feel that the drugs help you to get through. I expect you must wish for a time where you didn't feel so sad and bad about yourself?'
    'Yeah, sometimes.'
    'Hmm, so I wonder what kind of place you'd like to be in a few years' time?'
    'Well, I've always enjoyed painting, music and dance, and I used to be quite good at it. I never have a chance to do it now.'
    'How come?'
    'Well, it takes most of my time and energy to get money for the drugs, and when I'm high I don't feel the urge to paint, and I'd probably be crap at it if I did.'

This is an example of discrepancy. Once we discover it, we can start encouraging our patients to think about small steps on the way to narrowing the gap between where they would like to be and where they are now. It is not that we are forgetting about the addiction, it's more that we are helping them move along the process of change (*in Louise's case from pre-contemplation to contemplation of change*). But we are not making that case for them. It's important that they come up with their own chain of reasoning.

'Well, that must feel quite frustrating for you. How do you feel when you are painting?'
    'Well, it's amazing. Like, mostly, my head is always spinning and rushing. But when I'm painting, my head seems to go quiet, and other parts of me come out.'
    'Yes, I know that feeling. Have you ever thought of how you could find more time and head-space to do some more painting?'
    'Well, I guess I'd need to get rid of my shitty boyfriend. All he's interested in is sex and getting more money for Charlie.'

We are now at the stage where Louise can see personal reasons for change, and has identified something that she believes in. So we can start to talk about whether she currently has the self-efficacy (strength, energy and self-belief) to carry out a change. If she has, that's great. If not, we need to see what we can do to try to boost it.

'But won't it be hard to split up?'

'No, not really. He's a tosser and I'm only with him out of habit.'

'Well, I've known you a while, and I've always been impressed by your feisty spirit!'

'Yeah, although I can think of some people who might call me other names worse than that!'

'Like who?'

'Only most of the wankers I hang around with. They think I'm just a piece of shit.'

'Hmm, that's tough. Is there some way you can spend more time with people who are more supportive.'

'Well, my little sister has her own place now, and she's been asking for me to move back with her. Only I've been worried as I don't want her getting wrapped up in my shit.'

'Yes, that's a point. How would you feel about talking it through with her?'

'I guess that won't do any harm. I might go round later on.'

The aims appears to be to try to guide the patient towards achievable goals, as success breeds confidence. When our patients start to come up with achievable goals, we can start to gently explore and support their strategies, express optimism and give encouragement.

Activity 13.2: Motivating a patient

The next time you see a patient who needs a bit of motivating, consider what you will actually do to help them change, using some the tips suggested above:

- trying to avoid judgement
- building trust and rapport
- using 'change questions'
- rolling with any negative reactions
- looking for and exploring discrepancy
- helping build the patient's strength and 'efficacy' for change.

Be Drunk

Be drunk.

You have to be always drunk. That's all there is to it—it's the
  only way. So as not to feel the horrible burden of time that
  breaks your back and bends you to the earth, you have to
  be continually drunk.

But on what?

Wine, poetry or virtue . . . as you wish.

But be drunk.

And if sometimes, on the steps of a palace or the green grass
  of a ditch, in the mournful solitude of your room, you wake
  again, drunkenness already diminishing or gone, ask the
  wind, the wave, the star, the bird, the clock, everything
  that is flying, everything that is groaning, everything that
  is rolling, everything that is singing, everything that is
  speaking . . . ask what time it is and wind, wave, star, bird,
  clock will answer you: 'It is time to be drunk! So as not to
  be the martyred slaves of time, be drunk, be continually
  drunk!

On wine, on poetry or on virtue as you wish.'

– Charles Baudelaire

INTEGRATING MOTIVATIONAL COMMUNICATION INTO OUR PRACTICE

Motivational communicating is not the neutral communication we have discussed in other chapters. Motivating (like hypnosis) means trying to get our patients to move in a particular direction that we perceive is in their 'best interests', even when they might not entirely agree with us.

As we will discuss more in book 5, telling patients what they 'ought' to do is a form a 'moral judgement' that has no logical connection to our scientific and technical knowledge and training. We are very often unaware of our own bias, prejudice and ignorance, so making 'ought' statements from a position of power to patients who are vulnerable is an endeavour that is fraught with moral hazard. Thus, motivational interviewing requires a realisation and acceptance that there is a role for at least a degree of paternalism/maternalism in practice.

Not everyone will feel comfortable with this.

However, if we value the health of our patients, and recognise that, quite often, the biggest barrier to the patient's health is the patient themselves, we may be called into a situation of role conflict, for example between our role as 'trusted counsellor' (or as 'patient-centred' practitioner, or as 'non-judgemental practitioner') and our role as 'health promoter'.

To practise righteously in this situation requires that we try to gain our patients' consent, wherever that is possible, even if it is just consent from them for us to act paternalistically.

Despite the position of considerable strength, power and control we occupy as practitioners, and despite the terrible position of despair and collapse that some of our patients find themselves in, it is difficult to justify trying to manipulate covertly our patients' beliefs and actions.

Therefore, perhaps more than any other form of co-creation, we need to be mindful and self-aware before we start to use these more manipulative techniques. We need to remember that we too are subject to subconscious drives and motivations, and to acting out certain maladaptive dramas and narratives. We cannot fully escape these.

On the other hand, if pure motivation was the prerequisite for health practice there would be no health practitioners.

However, we can at least try to be aware of how we might be manipulating the patient for our own ends, rather than theirs.

The only sure way to find out how much we are manipulating, or how much consent our patients give us to manipulate them, is to check back with them. This means communicating effectively, both internally (recognising and interrogating our drives and narratives) and externally (ensuring the patient is aware of what we are trying to do, how we are trying to do it, and how to draw it to a close when they have had enough).

If patients do consent, and accept us with our flaws, we can start to determine what our commitment looks like, how effective that commitment is likely to be, and in which ways we can help our patients build both their commitment, but also their capacity, their efficacy, to change.

If we can achieve this 'well enough', we can start acting out of compassion for our patients, skilfully integrating the flow of information and communication between ourselves and our patients in ways that enable both patient and practitioner to get a clearer idea of where the 'ill health' is located; how best 'better health' can be co-created; and what steps the patient feels able to take on the road to creating that 'better' health. For desire is a very strong opponent, and sometimes only overcome by an even stronger desire in a different direction.

The Will to Win

If you want a thing bad enough
To go out and fight for it,
Work day and night for it,
Give up your time and your peace and
your sleep for it
If only desire of it
Makes you quite mad enough
Never to tire of it,
Makes you hold all other things tawdry
and cheap for it
If life seems all empty and useless without it
And all that you scheme and you dream is about it,
If gladly you'll sweat for it,
Fret for it, Plan for it,
Lose all your terror of God or man for it,
If you'll simply go after that thing that you want.
With all your capacity,
Strength and sagacity,
Faith, hope and confidence, stern pertinacity,
If neither cold poverty, famished and gaunt,
Nor sickness nor pain
Of body or brain
Can turn you away from the thing that you want,
If dogged and grim you besiege and beset it,
You'll get it!

— Berton Braley[84]

Chapter 14
Deciding

Activity 14.1: Good and bad decisions (30 minutes)

Allow your mind to wander back over the last few weeks. No doubt you have made many, many decisions as part of your practice.

In how many of these were you certain: most, about half, few, even fewer?

Choose some of the ones you were least certain about. What influenced your decisions? Try to itemise the various factors and influences.

How much did the patient concerned know about your uncertainty? How effective might it have been to involve them more?

Playing, storytelling, dancing, playing, modelling, acting and ritualising are all very well, but we are not paid to have fun. Sooner or later we have to make some decisions.

WHAT IS A GOOD DECISION?

As we go about co-creating healthier states of existence with our patients, sooner or later we have to make some decisions about what directions to take, what tools to use, and what outcomes we are looking for. The process of shared decision making is therefore a crucial one for health practice.

We all wish to make good decisions, but what is it that makes a good decision 'good'?[85]

A good decision may be something that achieves something that is most 'valuable' to us, or that is most 'useful', or perhaps the most 'effective'. What appears 'good' may be affected by the way we ask the question, or how we feel on the day, or by how we look at the world.

In short, a good decision can mean many things to many different people.[86] What appears to be a good decision to me may look quite like a bad decision to you.

Which is not surprising. What is 'good' anyway?

HEALTH DECISION MAKING

Health decision making is even more fraught with problems.

Health decisions are usually much more important to us than, say, the brand of ketchup or cola that we prefer,[87] so we tend to pay them special attention. But, again, what is 'good' health to me, may not look like 'good' health to you. And if we are feeling unwell, our capacity to make 'good' decisions, or even to want to make any decisions at all, may be affected.

Therefore one of our most important jobs as practitioners is to try to help patients come to 'good' decisions.

Unfortunately, we are just as prone to partiality, bias, prejudice or ignorance as the next person and no more likely to be 'objective' either.[88]

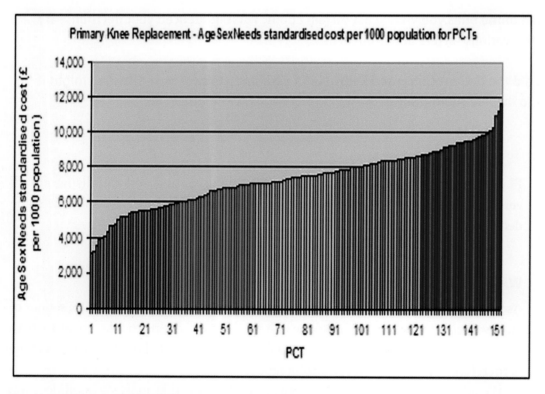

This graph, taken from the UK Department of Health 'Shared Decision Making' website, shows the huge geographical variation in knee replacement surgery across the UK, even though the rates of osteoarthritis are similar across the regions.[90]

Even if we are able to be objective, we are still in very muddy waters, because health is a highly complex and relational entity. That means that predicting outcomes and choosing options is a very complicated and inaccurate business. Even if we can find 'good' hard data (which as we will see in workbook 3 is not always in 'good' supply), we may not be that 'good' at understanding what the 'good' application of that evidence means in practice.

> I may think a treatment that reduces my relative risk of stroke by 50% sounds like an excellent idea, but may be less keen when I am told it only reduces my absolute risk by 1% (e.g. from 2% to 1%).[89]

As all bookmakers and gamblers will tell us, the practical application of probability is not an easy skill to acquire, let alone apply in such a sensitive area as one's own health. Perhaps for these reasons, we find that many health decisions vary from place to place and person to person, without any obvious logical reason. This has a significant impact, especially where potentially harmful or very expensive treatments are being used.

SHARED DECISION MAKING

We are obliged by the Hippocratic Oath to 'do no harm'. Because our patients are responsible for themselves, and because we can't always tell in advance if our suggestions may turn out to be harmful, we are also obliged to offer our patients an opportunity to share decisions about their healthcare. This is basic ethical practice.

But there are other 'good' practical reasons for shared decision making. Shared decisions appear to be more likely than practitioners' decisions to reduce unnecessary treatments, to improve concordance with care, to improve the quality of care, to increase satisfaction (for both patients and medical staff), to improve patients' self-esteem, to improve clinical safety, to reduce unwarranted practice variation, and to reduce litigation costs.[91]

Of course, not every patient wants to share decisions, and some prefer to ask their practitioner to decide on their behalf.[92] I'm not sure if this is paternalistic or patient-centred. Consider the following dialogue.

> *Doctor:* 'You need treatment X.'
> *Patient:* 'Anything you say doctor. I put myself in your hands.'

Perhaps paternalism versus patient-centredness is another false dichotomy?

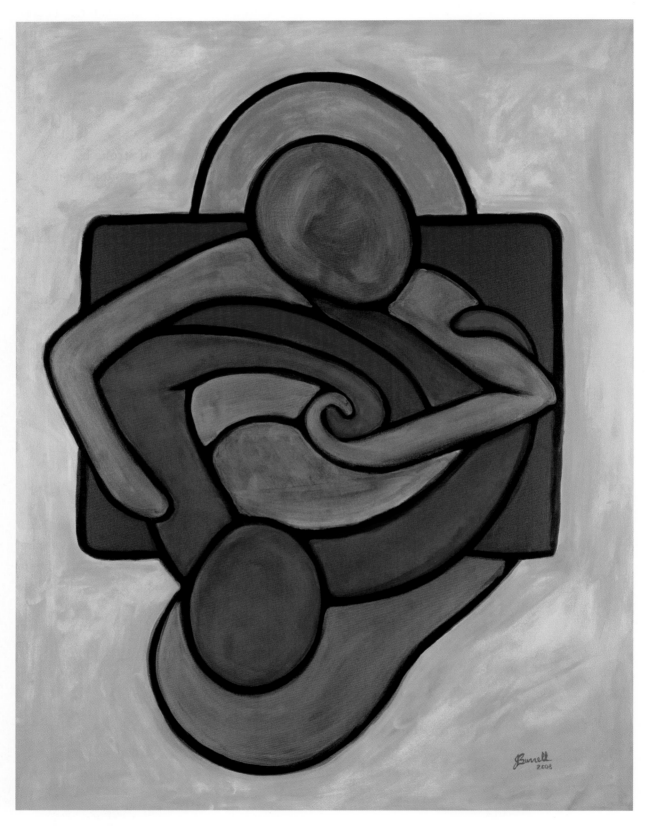

'Table Talk' – by Juliana Burrell[93]

INTEGRATING SHARED DECISION MAKING IN PRACTICE

'Good' shared decision making can be tricky in practice, for a number of 'good' pragmatic reasons. It takes time, there may be too many decisions to cover, patients may not feel well enough to engage, the available data may be inaccurate or patchy, or we may not know how to go about achieving a shared decision.[94]

For all these reasons, sometimes we have to prioritise those decisions where sharing can be most relevant and most effective.[95] The evidence suggests these would include decisions where there are several possible treatment approaches, where interventions may be risky, where there are significant cultural or subcultural differences between patient and practitioner and where the treatment will involve a lot of patient input or close concordance with difficult treatments.

As with any shared process, a sensible first step may be to check that everyone actually wants to be involved. As patients may not feel assertive enough to tell us they want to be involved, it is probably wiser simply to ask them.

> For example: 'People are all quite different. Some people like to know everything and be involved in the decisions, some people like to hand over to the practitioner, and some like to decide as they go along. Any of these approaches is OK with me. Which do you prefer?'

Perhaps the next step would be to try to determine the values, ideas, concerns and expectations of the patient and compare these with our own. This stage may take quite a lot of time and effort, but it is probably very important, particularly if our patient is from a different socioeconomic, cultural, age or ethnic group to ourselves. If we are not able to find common ground it is unlikely we will be able to create a management plan that works for both of us.

> Sometimes it is helpful to make these kind of rules explicit, for example: 'People have many different ideas about health and treatment, and that includes you and me. It's OK if these are different, but we should find out if and how so we can work with the differences as we develop the treatment plan?'

In trying to come to a shared decision, we hope to try to find out as much pertinent information as possible, and (as importantly) in a form that is accessible and understandable, both for our patients and ourselves.

Fortunately, there are now many sources of information, patient experience videos and diaries, health trainers and decision support tools that have been developed to help patients decide.[96]

As we all know, coming up with grand plans for our co-creations is one thing. Putting these plans into action and actually making the co-creation happen is another thing altogether. Success depends a great deal on how much belief and confidence we have in ourselves. When we are unwell, we tend to have much lower self-efficacy when we feel well and full of energy. It seems sensible therefore to start by making an assessment of the self-efficacy of both our patients and of ourselves. If either seems lacking, it may be wise to hold off decision making until it can be improved.

We can, however, help our patients (and colleagues) to improve self-efficacy in a number of ways. Primarily, we can model it. We can also ensure we set targets that they can reach, so they build confidence as they go. We can encourage and persuade them that that they can succeed. We can roll with ups and downs of emotions and moods, allowing them but not allowing them to dominate.

Many grand plans fail because of the detail. So we might wish to spend a little time imagining and thinking through each stage of the process, and considering factors that might unhinge success. These are the big and little things that are going to decide whether our decision will be effective or ineffective.[97]

Perhaps the biggest hurdle will be the availability of resources: time, money, facilities and, above all, our own personal resilience and efficacy. If we set the bar too high, we won't clear it. So we have to be realistic and accept that good enough is good enough.

However, if we keep perspective, we have reasons to be cheerful. Shared decision making may require more time and energy at the outset, but in the longer term one of the upsides of shared decision making is that the practitioner does not have to make all the running. This is where the great value of shared decision making becomes apparent for practitioners as well as patients.

Effective shared decision making involves recruiting the patient as an ally, and using his or her resources to do the some of the homework. If we can be mindful enough, and aware enough, to see the value of dedicating a little more time and energy up front, the payback is that we may find our patients are much more involved in, and effective at, managing their own care, and co-creating healthier states of existence.

What the Doctor Said

He said it doesn't look good

he said it looks bad in fact real bad

he said I counted thirty-two of them on one lung before

I quit counting them

I said I'm glad I wouldn't want to know

about any more being there than that

he said are you a religious man do you kneel down

in forest groves and let yourself ask for help

when you come to a waterfall

mist blowing against your face and arms

do you stop and ask for understanding at those moments

I said not yet but I intend to start today

he said I'm real sorry he said

I wish I had some other kind of news to give you

I said Amen and he said something else

I didn't catch and not knowing what else to do

and not wanting him to have to repeat it

and me to have to fully digest it

I just looked at him

for a minute and he looked back it was then

I jumped up and shook hands with this man who'd just

 given me

something no one else on earth had ever given me

I may have even thanked him habit being so strong

– Raymond Carver[98]

Activity 14.2: Integrating shared decision making in practice (1 hour)

There are now numerous resources to aid practitioners and patients make shared decisions. Spend some time browsing through some of them, or discover others, and try using some of them this week, with two or three patients.

- Health Talk Online at www.healthtalkonline.org/Improving_health_care/shared_decision_making

- National Prescribing Centre Decision Aids at www.npc.nhs.uk/evidence/eidm4_shared/pda.php

- University of Sydney Decision Aids at http://sydney.edu.au/medicine/public-health/shdg/resources/decision_aids.php

- Right Care (part of the NHS) at www.rightcare.nhs.uk/index.php/shared-decision-making

- The Informed Medical Decisions Foundation at http://informedmedicaldecisions.org/shared-decision-making-in-practice/decision-aids

Conclusion – integrating the 'we' relationship

When we meet another person, we communicate instantly and automatically; seeing, hearing, touching, smelling, listening, speaking, dancing, singing, acting, transferring, storytelling, playing and even ritualising. But despite the fact that we use so many different forms of communication, we only have one integrated experience. That is because our consciousness integrates that communication and 'creates' our experience, in a seamless, balanced and integrated whole.

In the 'we' relationship, there are always at least two conscious beings; both of whom create. I create you as you create me, and we create ourselves and each other. That co-creation is what we experience and it is *all* we experience.

If we can only 'know' each other through the lens of our co-creation, it follows that, the more clouded and confused the 'we' co-creation is, the harder it will be for us, as practitioners, to discover and be able to act upon important information we are receiving and giving.

For all these reasons, perspective is crucial. In an infinite and relational universe, there are an infinite number of perspectives. Complexity and uncertainty are everywhere. But there is also unity. There is only one thing that we experience, and that one thing is everything we experience. So it is probably wise to try to find out from our patients what that experience is, for them.

As practitioners, we have available a wealth of information about our patients: from sense data, from technology, from speaking and listening, and from the whole range of non-verbal communication that we use. If we are to be integrated practitioners, we hope to be able to become aware of, analyse, and apply as much of this information as we can.

> It is not that we wish to be skilful scientists *or* skilful communicators. We wish to be both.

The advance of empirical and technological forms of communication has opened up possibilities in classification, pathology, diagnosis, investigation, treatment, training and management that we could not have dreamt of 200 years ago. These are valuable advances. Even if we wanted to, we cannot turn back the clock. Science, empiricism and technology will remain an integral part of health practice. We are left with no choice except to value and use these tools, albeit skilfully.

The advance of the understanding and practice of interpretive and intuitive models of communication has shown that we are, perhaps above all, communicators. We live in, and cannot step out of, the rich, deep and complex web of stories, games, dances, songs, dramas and rituals of our shared human interaction. Objectivity is an aspiration long gone. We are left with no choice except to value and use these tools, albeit skilfully.

> **From one perspective, we *are* communication of information, because the whole universe is an interplay of information. Everything is that one thing.**

In using communication, we communicate with all of ourselves in one go, consciously and subconsciously. Contrary to the theoretical terminology we have fallen into the sloppy habit of using, in practice we cannot separate out our 'conscious' and 'unconscious'; our 'sensory' and 'interpretive' approaches.

Thoughts, ideas and emotions arise spontaneously, within our imaginations and without a tag that explains where they come from. We co-create with our patients in a very powerful, complex and interrelated way, so it is therefore very easy to get sidetracked and to lose track of whose emotions and experiences belong to whom.

Therefore, being an effective and integrated practitioner suggests trying to cultivate a deep, compassionate intimacy and empathy with oneself.

From that starting point we may communicate more effectively with ourselves, and learn more about ourselves. As we become more self-aware, we may learn to detach ourselves from those elements of our existence which are unbalanced or ineffective or unskilful. As we learn to detach we can learn to still and to clear our minds, and enter the 'we' relationship in a state of poised, peaceful, clear-minded awareness. From there we will be able to communicate, assess and act far more quickly, effectively and efficiently.

If we go into communication with our patients when we are feeling irritable, or distracted, angry, anxious or bored; we will not know how to interpret those emotions if they re-emerge while we are with the patient.[99] We will quite literally get back what we put in. Our co-creation will be negative, and ineffective, and, perhaps most importantly, almost impossible to use therapeutically.

Communication is probably the nearest thing to miracle that we experience. Familiarity may have bred contempt, but the idea that, through sights, sounds and gestures, we can open up the rich complexity of our existences to each other is astonishing, almost impossible to believe.

It is as if at some point the universe just told two handfuls of dust to get up and start discussing the weather. We would not believe that could happen. But it did. And we do.

Through our communication we don't just 'witness' the existence of our partner, we actually experience that existence for ourselves, through the medium of our co-creation. That experience gives us a unique and incredible insight into what it is to be our patients, and it gives our patients a unique and incredible insight into what it is to be us.

If what our patient experiences through their insight into us is a practitioner who appears compassionate, courageous and honest; we have the best chance of our patients beginning to speak in an honest and forthright way, which gives us even further insight into them, and vice versa.

In practical terms, giving our patients just one minute, without interruption, in which they can express themselves, while we watch and listen in complete absorption; may be the most important, effective and efficient health practice skill we can learn.

What then arises is a whole palette of colours, from which we can pick and choose to paint our co-creation in any way we want, through using every bit of ourselves. It is not just a technical process, though it is a technical process. It is complete expression in which we can choose to touch, see, hear, think, feel, sing, narrate, transfer, model, ritualise, dance and even play.

As we dance (or sing, or play . . .) together, we pull all these various threads of information together within our imagination, and using that imagination we co-create a new existence within which we get ever greater and more accurate insight into each other, and from which we can build ever more possibility for healing.

Insight illuminates darkness, listening fosters understanding, and speaking helps dispel the seeds of darkness and despair. That is the virtuous cycle that lies at the heart of effective practice, and at the heart of effective self-practice.

The Healer
Seeing
Hearing
Touching
Feeling

Imagine

Thinking
Sharing
Holding
Caring

Healing

– JA

Activity: Co-Create with a friend (as long as you need)

Choose a friend. Go and have some fun.

Co-create something special . . .

You deserve it.

Notes

1 The clue is in the title. Practitioners tend to be practical. While we might like to know the theory behind what we do, what tends to be more important is that it works. The original 'Integrated Practitioner' is a whole work comprising both theory and practice. This series of workbooks is intended to be more practical, so in books 1–4 the practice will predominate. For those that are interested, the fifth workbook, *Food for Thought*, will discuss more of the theory that lies behind this work, as of course does the original book.

However, for now, please bear with us, as there are 13 key theoretical points that underpin this work and without which it may not make complete sense. They are as follows.

1. The universe, and every-'thing' within it, came into existence from no-'thing', and may presumably go back into nothing, and we can say nothing about the nothing, as there is nothing to say.

2. The universe and everything within it (including ourselves) is entirely and intrinsically relational. Within this relational web, certain states of matter and energy 'exist' (stand out) with varying degrees of complexity (entropy) against that background of nothingness.

3. Complex entities in the universe are holarchical. This means each level of complexity creates a whole which is greater than the sum of the parts. So, for example, clusters of atoms create molecules, clusters of molecules create cells, clusters of cells create organs, clusters of organs create beings, and clusters of beings create cultures and societies and biospheres. Each one of these can be said to exist on its own, as the interplay of smaller parts, and as part of the greater whole.

4. Fascinatingly, and slightly disturbingly, we find that things that may appear to us to be fixed are also relational. These include knowledge, truth, beliefs, meanings and eventually health itself. Not only are they relational, they are also self-referential. For example, truth is a function of meaning, meaning is a function of language, and language is a function of truth. Self-referential systems always end up in paradox. It is therefore impossible to define with certainty what 'health' is.

5. The universe is made up of the interplay between three things: forces, energy and matter. However, our experience of the universe is far, far richer than that. We feel warmth, beauty, taste, colour and texture. We experience anger, hope, fear, courage, joy and love. The reason that the universe appears so much richer to us is because of our consciousness. Consciousness takes in cold sense data derived from the forces, energy and matter of the universe, and uses them to

create the full richness of our existence. In other words, and in a very real way, our consciousness creates itself, and creates our experience of existence, as we go along.

6. While we think ourselves as having independent, concrete identity, this is actually just a matter of perspective. From a more macroscopic perspective, we are one infinitesimally small part of much larger relational systems: for example, our societies, our cultures, the biosphere, the noosphere, and the cosmos. From a microscopic perspective each one of our molecules and atoms comes from somewhere (or someone) else and goes somewhere (or to someone) else. From a quantum perspective we exist at the level of probability. From a cultural perspective the words, ideas and beliefs we use are mostly given to us by others.

7. When two conscious persons come into relationship with each other, each person's consciousness creates both itself and the other person. In other words, in relating to each other, in a very real way, we co-create each other.

8. Time does not flow. It is simply part of the space–time continuum. Our sense of time flowing derives from two things. First, our memory links together different states of existence in the space–time continuum in a linear way, giving us the idea that past flows into present. Second, our consciousness imagines future states of existence, giving us the idea that present flows into future.

9. This ability of consciousness to create past, present and future; to create itself; and to co-create others clearly has profound implications for what we think of as health, ill-health and health practice.

10. Health does not exist outside consciousness. It is a relational truth created by individuals, cultures and societies that has different meanings when viewed from different perspectives (for example, biomedical, psychological, sociological, or spiritual perspectives).

11. A common theme emerging from these different perspectives appears to be that health is something to do with the attainment and maintenance of a harmonic balance between different relational entities (for example, between molecules, between cells, between organs, between mind and body, between people, or between groups and societies).

12. While we cannot say what health is, we can suggest that health practice can therefore be seen as an attempt to co-create and maintain a harmonic, relational balance, not just for our patients but also for ourselves and our societies.

13. Being an integrated practitioner involves integrating all of the relationships and perspectives of our shared existence, using all of the tools that we have created and evolved through the history of human existence, to co-create 'healthier' states of existence from 'less healthy' states of existence. Health practice is therefore a science and a technology, but it is also fundamentally creative and therefore artistic.

That is enough of the theory. Let's get practical. After all, we are practitioners not theorists.

2 Edward Henry Potthast (1857–1927): 'Along the Mystic River'. Public domain art.

3 'Ars Poetica' by Archibald MacLeish, from *Collected Poems, 1917–1982*, Boston:

Houghton Mifflin; 1985. ISBN: 0395394171. Reprinted with kind permission of the Houghton Mifflin Company.

4   We don't just exist as entities. We exist as *self-conscious* entities. That gives us a whole new set of existences at different levels and perspectives of our consciousness. We are not just conscious. We are also *conscious of being conscious*, and conscious of being conscious of being conscious (and so on and so on).

5   We can communicate in different ways because we exist in different ways. First, we exist at different levels. Each level is whole and complete, but made up of lower levels, and is part of yet higher levels. These levels are known as 'holons' (*see* workbook 5 for more discussion of this). For example, we exist as atoms, molecules, cells, genes, organs, physiological systems and as conscious individuals. Our existence doesn't stop there. We also exist as members of families, peer groups, organisations, societies and cultures. Ultimately, we exist as a part of the biosphere and as a part of the universe as a whole. Within our consciousness we merge and integrate numerous sources and types of information: sense data, memories, emotions, feelings, ideas, fears, hopes, words, thoughts and so on. So although we often refer to our mind as 'one thing', it is more like a collective term that we use to describe all the voices, perspectives, thoughts, beliefs and emotions that we hold, either consciously or subconsciously, at any one time.

6   For example, we may start talking about 'subconscious' versus 'conscious' communication; or 'physical' versus 'psychological'; or 'practical' versus 'ideal', or 'conceptual' versus 'phenomenological' or 'verbal' versus 'non-verbal'. These distinctions can be useful tools if they help us to unpick, analyse and then reintegrate our practice. For example, in the table below we can look at different forms of communication and relate them to different levels of our existence. However, these distinctions can also be tyrants. We may wish to take great care with them in case we get sucked into the illusion that they actually exist. To try to avoid that, we may ask ourselves some tricky questions such as:

   • Where does my 'subconscious' start, and my 'conscious' begin?
   • Could we have a 'psychological' existence without a 'physical' one; or vice versa?
   • What are 'ideas' and 'concepts' if not the product of 'phenomenological' interaction between our 'physical' natures and our 'conceptual' natures?
   • Is it possible to have an 'idea' that is not tied in some way to a 'practical' experience, or vice versa?

   As we will see in this book, communication is not easily bounded or limited by simple distinctions and divisions. When we communicate, we do so in an integrated and whole way, and we have an integrated and whole sense of that communication.

7   All of these levels, entities and relationalities make it very difficult for us to pin down who exactly we are, and this has been a question which scientists and philosophers continue to wrestle with today. Many theorists have tried to classify and grade many of these different levels of existence. These theoretical debates seem to generate much heat, but not a great deal of light. 'Classical' philosophers tended to suggest that we have a real existence and that change to that existence is incidental. 'Process philosophers' (such as Albert North Whitehead) argue the opposite: that change *is* who we are, and that any concept of concrete existence is illusory. Western

religions tend to teach the existence of the soul as the centre of existence of the self; Eastern religions tend to teach the non-existence of the self. Materialists (such as some Marxian and Scientific Materialists) argue that our existence is entirely material (i.e. physical); whereas idealists (such as Hegel and Berkeley) suggest we only exist as our ideas of our own existence. Dualists (such as Descartes) argue we are both material and ideal. Wilber makes the interesting point that how we appear to be is a matter of perspective. We will create what we appear to be by the way we choose to see ourselves (i.e. if we use physical tools to see ourselves we will appear physical, and if we use conceptual tools we will appear conceptual). Fortunately, we are practitioners not theorists, so we can leave classifications and definitions to one side, and concentrate on techniques and skills that seem to work in practice.

8   Simon and Garfunkel. *The Sounds of Silence*, Columbia – CS 9269. Released 1965.

9   As soon as we come into contact with any other person, we gather a great deal of information about how they look (from their overall demeanour to small particularities about the way they hold themselves, their gait, their choice of clothing or hairstyle and so on); how they smell (both consciously and through subconscious pheromonal activity); what they sound like (the tone and character of their voice, their breathing, the sound of their gait); and what they feel like (dry, puffy, spongy, hairy, scaly etc.).

10   The word 'sign' can mean many different things to many different people. In the medical world, it tends to mean an observable correlate of an underlying 'disease' (which sets it apart from 'symptoms' which are the subjective experiences of the condition as described by the patient). However, signs can be many other things too. They can be metaphors which symbolise meaningful concepts; they help us classify and categorise; they help us develop meaning, belonging and narrative; and of course they are forms of communication (for what are words if not signs?).

11   For example, pain causes activity in the 'autonomic' nervous system that we are all aware of, such as pallor, sweating, muscle tension, physical withdrawal, crying and moaning. Liver failure causes yellow discolouration of the skin, flapping hands, weight loss, swollen abdomen, and 'drunken' gait. There are many more of these correlates, which form 'patterns' which we are trained to spot as practitioners. The more patients we see, the more we automate recognition of these patterns, eventually finding ourselves able to 'spot-diagnose' patients as they walk into the room.

12   'Signs' by Osnat Tzadok. More of Osnat's work can be found at her websites at www.osnatfineart.com and www.OsnatGreetingCards.com

13   Sensing and intuition describe the way we perceive, gather and interpret information. Initially, we sense the data as raw data, then we try to match it to pre-existing cognitive scripts or patterns, and finally we attempt to make linkages between the information and other memorised or observed information. This final stage is what gives 'meaning' to the information. Myers-Briggs personality theory suggests that we all have preferences towards either of these two dialectical positions. Those of us who prefer 'sensing' prefer to build the information carefully from the bottom up, arriving at meaning only once the foundations have been laid. Those of us who prefer 'intuition' prefer to match and interpret data quickly, then use our senses to try to backfill and cross check the interpretation. Commonly, intuits will accuse

sensors of paralysis by analysis, whereas sensors will accuse intuits of irresponsible leaps to unjustified conclusions!

14 For example, breast cancer screening saves 1400 lives a year in England (Durojave 2009). Smallpox has been eradicated. Screening and examination of pregnant women has led to significant reductions in maternal and infant mortality. We can now carry out lower risk and more effective treatments, for example angiographic treatment of ischaemic heart disease and targeted radiotherapy.

15 Patients diagnosed with hypertension take more sick leave, have more marital problems and score lower on self-rated health and quality of life scores, and take longer to recover from other illnesses (Ogedegbe 2010).

16 Harms from screening include: complications arising from the investigation; unnecessary effects of treatment; unnecessary treatment of persons with inconsequential disease; adverse effects of stigma and labelling; costs and inconvenience incurred during investigations and treatment; and consequences of false-negative results. False-negative results may cause harms from delays in diagnosis and treatment, false reassurance, loss of confidence in practitioners, legal and economic costs. False positives may cause distress and harms from further testing, unnecessary treatments, costs and complications. Screening programmes as a whole are expensive and may make social health inequalities worse. The numbers needed to screen to prevent one death over 10 years is 1173 for colorectal cancer and 500 for breast cancer.

However, the cumulative risk of false positives for mammograms may be up to 49%. Therefore it is possible that, in some screening programmes, more people may be harmed than benefit from that screening programme. We now have screening tests for many cancers (e.g. breast, bowel, cervical, prostate and ovarian). If we look at all screening programmes for all these cancers together, the risk of false positive increases further (for 3 years' worth of screening the probability of false positives is 60% for men and 49% for women, and the risk of undergoing harmful procedures is 29% for men and 22% for women) (US National Cancer Institute 2012).

17 King 1982.

18 Words are units of meaning that translate 'my' thoughts into 'your' thoughts, and vice versa. Because we cannot 'see' each other's internal worlds, we have to do the next best thing, which is to translate our thoughts into words and sentences and express them to our listener, who has to translate our words into thoughts in their own mind. Words are therefore (arguably) our most powerful tool. However, there be dragons . . .

- We are not aware of all our thoughts, as some are subconscious.
- It is not possible to select, translate and express all those thoughts that we are aware of as there are too many.
- The selection process we use to choose which thoughts to translate and transmit is subconsciously influenced by our subconscious.
- We may be unable to find words which exactly and accurately express our thoughts.
- We miss a lot of what is said to us.
- Those words we do hear may mean something different to us than to the speaker.

- What we hear isn't the same as what we understand, as subconscious factors may influence our interpretation.

19 Please see the 'Cambridge Calgary Guide' (in Kurtz, Silverman & Draper 2005) for a fantastic review of all the evidence about communication skills in practice. In summary, poor communication is associated with worse patient understanding, worse patient outcomes, worse adherence to treatment, higher costs, worse response to treatment, and increased litigation.

20 Doctors interrupt on average only 17 seconds after the patient starts talking. However, if patients are allowed to talk uninterrupted, they will usually finish what they want to say with 90 seconds. If a doctor interrupts early we miss over half the patient's concerns, the consultation is more likely to be dysfunctional, we are more likely to misdiagnose and mistreat our patients, and the consultation is likely to take longer. (Kurtz, Silverman & Draper 2005).

21 Deep listening suggests absolute presence and awareness on the part of the listener, who pays close attention, without interrupting or distracting the speaker, and listens for both verbal and non-verbal communication. It is active as well. Deep listening involves summarising and checking back to ensure correct understanding and interpretation. Ultimately, deep listening is not just an attempt to understand the communication; it is an attempt to experience what it is **to be** the other person. Therefore deep listening is also a form of creative imagination.

22 Simple 'person-centred' non-directive counselling has been the subject of much research. It is an extremely difficult area to research, as there are many confounding variables (counselling by one counsellor in one location with one patient using one approach may be extremely different to a different counsellor/location/approach/ patient). Also, the possible outcome measures cannot really capture the full complexity of what it is to 'feel', let alone what it is to 'feel better' (*see* Introduction for a fuller discussion of this). However, such evidence as there is suggests that counselling is effective for mild to moderate mental health problems, as effective as antidepressants, although neither seem to make a huge difference in the long term (or if they do the effect is lost in an ocean of confounding variables). For a good review of the evidence look at *Effectiveness Matters: counselling in primary care*. (NHS Centre for Reviews 2001).

23 Again, have a look at Kurtz, Silverman & Draper (2005) for more detail, but a wealth of evidence shows doctors interrupt too soon, use closed questions, grossly overestimate how much time we give to explaining, focus our explanations on our own agenda (i.e. the treatment) rather than the patient's agenda, never get to the bottom of the patient's ideas, concerns and understandings (and therefore cannot tailor explanations to the patients ideas, concerns and understandings), use too much jargon, and fail to demonstrate empathy and understanding in our communication.

24 'Anger' from *Seven Deadly Sins, Anger* by Michael Craig-Martin born 1941, **Date:** 2008. Presented by the artist and Alan Cristea Gallery 2009. © Michael Craig-Martin. Reproduced by kind permission of the artist.

25 Useful CBT resources include the following.

- British Association for Behavioural & Cognitive Psychotherapies: www.babcp. com

- Beating the Blues: www.beatingtheblues.co.uk
- The 'Overcoming' series: www.overcoming.co.uk
- MoodGYM: information, quizzes, games and skills training to help prevent depression: www.moodgym.anu.edu.au
- Living Life to the Full: free online life skills course: www.llttf.com
- FearFighter: www.fearfighter.com
- Blenkiron P. *Stories and Analogies in Cognitive Behavioural Therapy*. Oxford: Wiley Blackwell; 2010.
- Williams CJ, Garland A. Cognitive-behavioural therapy assessment model for use in clinical practice. *Adv Psych Treat*. 2002; **8**: 172–79.
- DOH. *Improving Access to Psychological Therapies (IAPT) Programme: computerised Cognitive Behavioural Therapy (cCBT) implementation guidance*. Department of Health, UK; March 2007.
- National Institute for Health and Care Excellence. *Anxiety: management of anxiety (panic disorder, with or without agoraphobia, and generalised anxiety disorder) in adults in primary, secondary and community care*. NICE. March 2011.
- National Institute for Health and Care Excellence. *Cognitive Behavioural Therapy for the Management of Common Mental Health Problems*. NICE. December 2010.
- National Institute for Health and Care Excellence. *Computerised Cognitive Behaviour Therapy for Depression and Anxiety: review of Technology Appraisal 51*. NICE. February 2006.

26 Narrative therapy tries to help patients recognise, express and then develop (or 'thicken') stories that do not support or sustain problems. The idea is that patients start to live within and express healthier stories, so the stories become the launch pad for healthier self-creation.

Narrative therapy derives from a 'post-structuralist' philosophy. Structuralism is the idea that there are basic 'structures' to cultural, linguistic, sociological and psychological existence, wherever we come from or whoever we are. Structuralism therefore looks for and studies our 'basic' needs, motives, attributes, traits, strengths, deficits, resources, properties, characteristics, drives and so on.

Post-structuralism denies that these structures exist and, even if they did, it would be impossible to step outside these structures to describe or define them. Post-structuralism therefore looks instead for our intentions, purposes, values, beliefs, hopes, dreams, visions and commitments.

According to post-structuralism (and hence narrative therapy), each of our 'holons' (as individuals, families, cultures and societies) both derives from, and experiences our existence as, a complex relational web of stories or narratives that we tell each other and ourselves. The narratives we tell ourselves and each other spring from a highly complex relational set of entities which may include, but are not limited to, our cultures, our families, our training, our memories, our beliefs, our hopes, and so on.

As individuals, as families and as cultures we tell each other some narratives that are more or less dominant than others. This means that some narratives can become tyrannical, and others marginalised (even though the marginalised ones may be intrinsically healthier).

The key theme behind narrative therapy is that 'the person is not the problem'. It aims to deconstruct all the relevant narratives that the patients are using. By 'externalising' concerns or problems, patients can get an external perspective. Rather than identifying themselves with the problems, they begin to see that their problems can be dealt with separately and independently. By helping patients deconstruct and then reconstruct their own personal narratives into ones that are richer, more whole, and healthier; the patient can then become richer, more whole and healthier. Ultimately, the aim is to co-create alternative stories and possible directions that we can take, which are more integrated with our values, beliefs and aspirations.

The role of the practitioner within this perspective is that of the 'investigative reporter' who continuously asks questions of and challenges the stories we tell, always trying to help the patient bring the story 'out' where it can be critically analysed, deconstructed, reconstructed and then given its proper, balanced, integrated place within the host of other narratives with which and through which we exist. Sometimes the practitioner may ask others in to the consultation, so that they can 'witness' the other narratives or other perspectives on particular narratives. However, the practitioner does not take positions about, or judge, particular stories as being more or less healthy. The practitioner merely helps patients become aware of alternatives, and helps patients thicken those alternative narratives they choose.

This 'thickening' is important. Patients will find it difficult to live new narratives that are too thin and sketchy. So the practitioner spends time getting the patients to ensure the new narratives are as complex, rich and deep as possible; looking into how they will impact on all the different parts of the patients' lives. (White & Epston 1990; Greenhalgh & Hurwitz 2002; Launer 2002)

27 From *Life* magazine, 1943.

28 'Then and Now' by Oodgeroo of the tribe Noonuccal. From: Noonuccal, Oodgeroo. *My People*, 3rd ed. Milton, Queensland: The Jacaranda Press; 1990. Reproduced by permission of John Wiley & Sons Australia.

29 Outside the specific context of psychotherapy, where therapists can spend many hours working with clients, narrative therapy still has a role in other forms of practice. While we may not be able to go into the depth or breadth of specialised therapists, we can still use an approach where our style focuses on questions that make people think, rather than focusing on finding the answer. Probing, even challenging, questioning of the storyline, imagery, assumptions and style can be helpful in enabling patients see their problems from a more balanced perspective. This has become known as 'conversations inviting change'.

30 The stages of narrative therapy are broadly as follows.
   • Getting the patient to describe what is going on in their lives, listening very carefully to the stories they tell and the words and imagery they use to tell their stories.
   • Narrowing down to those problems that are most concerning or overwhelming. These are called 'problem-saturated stories'. The problem saturation can become so great that the stories can be taken on as actual identities. For example, we may hear ourselves define ourselves as a 'depressive', or as 'happy go lucky', or a 'worry-guts', or 'I'm hopeless').
   • Externalising the problem: by helping the patient to understand that they and

the problem are different things. So if someone says I am hopeless, we might ask whether they mean they are absolutely hopeless or that they have little hope, as these of course are different things entirely. We might ask the patient to give the problem an actual persona, and imagine it is sitting. Or we can ask patients to imagine a third party who knows them to try to describe what they see. Externalising the problem like this disempowers it, reduces guilt and blame, and opens new possibilities.

- Mapping the problem: once we have helped the patient identify and externalise the problem we can start to explore and map it. The idea is to understand how the problem story is actually experienced, then to understand the power, meaning and impact of the story; and then ask for evidence to support or undermine the power of the problem. We can use questions like: 'Is it true you are "always" depressed, or are there some times you feel more hopeful?' Or we can challenge imagery and metaphor. For example, if our patient says, 'I feel totally beaten by this,' we can ask them in what way this beating occurs, which part of them is beaten, who is the beater and what he uses to do the beating? All of these approaches can help patients see that their story is not necessarily saturated with problems, that their problems are not as powerful and pervasive as they might think, and that alternative stories may be possible. We don't need to take sides, or even comment upon the value of different stories. Rather we can just collaborate with our patients as they externalise and then explore the problems. We can act as detective, investigative reporter, historian or scientist.
- Looking for different, more positive outcomes: by asking questions like, 'Is it true you always feel hopeless?', or 'Is there ever a time when you don't feel hopeful' or, 'Would other people always see you as hopeless?' We can help patients to see that alternative stories, with more positive outcomes, are possible. Narrative therapists call these 'unique outcomes'.
- Re-authoring: once a new storyline is raised, it can start to be thickened up and re-authored. For example: what will it look like when you are like that? How might it support you?

31 'The Thin People' by Sylvia Plath, from *The Collected Poems* by Sylvia Plath, Faber and Faber; First US edition (2002). Reprinted with kind permission of Faber and Faber.

32 Hypnosis is not dissimilar to mindful awareness, and indeed mindful awareness is a form of hypnotic state. Both require the development of focused attention, concentration, detachment from other states and concerns, equanimity, acceptance, non-judgement, and mindful presence.

33 A good review of the evidence for hypnotherapy can be found in two Special Issues of the *International Journal of Clinical and Experimental Hypnosis* on 'Evidence-based practice in clinical hypnosis' (Various 2007). In brief the benefits of hypnosis seem to be greatest in anxiety disorders, pain management, distraction during unpleasant procedures, sleep disorders, 'psychosomatic' disorders and unwelcome habits; as well as for lifestyle and personal development goals such as performance in sports or work, public speaking and the creative arts. Hypnosis seems to be most effective when combined with a cognitive approach (*see* Chapter 3 'Singing').

34 Erickson wrote extensively about the subconscious mind, which he believed was a creative force, quite separate from, but in constant communication with, our conscious minds. He thought that we are always subconsciously open to new suggestion, and that we automatically 'allow' new suggestions to participate, or not participate, in subconscious communication. We enter trance states frequently, for example when our minds are switched off, when we are exercising, when we get interrupted in the middle of complex activities (such as tying shoelaces, or singing a song), when we are confronted with something amazing, or when we are struck by an idea or observation that is dissonant with our current understandings and beliefs. He also showed that these trance states have physical correlates, such as stillness, lateral eye movements, reduced respiration and heart rate, and a disconnection with the present.

   Rather than using specific trance induction, he showed how trances can be generated in everyday conversation so we can communicate with each other's unconscious minds without the other person knowing about it. However, he also taught that the subconscious does not respond to direct instruction, preferring instead more artful and metaphorical language, paradox and contradiction.

   He did this by a variety of techniques, including:
   - ambiguous language to create doubt and dissonance
   - 'artfully vague' language that leaves room for the patient to fill in the gaps
   - generation of confusion and dissonance by using meaningless sentences or dropping/deleting phrases or ending sentences abruptly
   - touch (particularly the 'hypnotic handshake' where the handshake starts in one way, pauses, and then takes on a different character)
   - the use of permissive instructions, such as you might feel you are becoming more relaxed.

35 Neurolinguistic programming is a therapeutic approach that draws on a number of different foundations: from hypnosis, through linguistics and social learning (modelling) to motivational approaches. The name comes from the idea that we process our experiences of reality through our neurological senses, interpret the sense data using internal linguistics (which gives the experiences meaning and structure), and then programme ourselves using the same linguistic systems (internally and externally) and thereby change our behaviours in an adaptive (or maladaptive) way.

   NLP is particularly interested in two related but separate cycles. The first is the interior conceptual cycle (sense data → neurological processing → ideas/thoughts/emotions → conceptual map → actions → sense data). The second is the behavioural cycle (experience → knowledge → action → experience). These two loops give us two different experiences of our existence: the internal conceptual 'map'; and the external, phenomenological 'territory'. One of the key themes of NLP is that the 'territory is not the map'; and the aim of therapy is often to develop our conceptual maps to become more accurate, more inclusive and more effective representations of the exterior territory of existence.

36 Erikson developed an extensive use of therapeutic metaphor and story as well as hypnosis and coined the term brief therapy for his approach of addressing therapeutic changes in relatively few sessions.

37 An 'anchor' is an NLP term for particular triggers which lead to particular emotional or behavioural states. It consists of both the trigger and the response. Anchors are therefore analogous to computer programs that execute once certain criteria are met, and thereafter run automatically, often below the level of awareness. Anchors can be adaptive (e.g. if they trigger us to jump out of the way when we hear a noise sounding like an onrushing train) or maladaptive (e.g. if they lead to us getting grumpy every time we feel hungry; or panicking every time we go into a supermarket). In practice, these often are presented as phobias, obsessions or compulsions. NLP approaches aim to help patients initially become aware of the anchors (bring them into consciousness), watch and monitor them to seek patterns and triggers; and then try reprogramming different, more healthy behavioural responses in reaction to the triggers (e.g. saying a comforting rhyme as you go into the supermarket to replace and distract from the previous anxious behaviours). Ultimately, it aims to 'collapse' maladaptive anchors completely, so that they no longer trigger unwanted reactions.

38 'After Apple Picking', Robert Frost, in *North of Boston*, published by Henry Holt and Co, 1953. Public domain poetry.

39 Non-verbal communications include the following.
- Facial expressions: these are probably the greatest source of non-verbal communication. They tell us about a person's identity, mood, sex, age, aggression, interest and much more. There is cultural variation (for example, in some countries smiling is a sign of friendliness, in others it's a sign of idiocy). Certain expressions seem fairly universal, for example anger, happiness and sadness. Some facial expressions are harder to distinguish, such as disgust and fear.
- Eye movements: we can convey meaning by opening or closing our eyes, by gazing in different directions, by the amount of time we make direct eye contact for, by how much we blink, and by the degree of pupil dilation (which may suggest aggression, attraction, boredom or interest).
- Gestures: gestures can be conscious, but more often they are subconscious, so again they provide powerful information to the listener. They may accentuate what we are saying, or provide additional information. For example, in health practice patients may use different hand gestures to describe different sorts of pain, which provide very useful diagnostic information. For example, I have noticed that patients often point with one or two fingers at their epigastrium when they have upper GI pain; with a flat palm over the centre when they have diffuse lower GI pain; or with clenched fists over their chests when they have angina or oesophageal spasm.
- Paralinguistics: we use vocal communications which are not words. We layer many other features onto the actual words we use, such as variations in tone, volume, accent, inflection and so on. Much of this is innate. However, we are very good at altering our voice with different people (think of how we talk to children). Whether we like it or not, through our voices we express our emotions and attitudes.
- Posture: If we lean forward towards someone it suggests interest, and the opposite

if we lean back. Crossing our arms and legs may suggest threat or frustration, whereas relaxed open gestures suggest relaxation.

- Space: the amount of space we like to have between ourselves and other people (proxemics), which varies with age, sex, culture, intimacy and type of conversation.
- Touch: touch is perhaps the first form of communication we use as newborn babies, and it remains a very intimate form through adult life: We may touch each other (e.g. handshaking, kissing, patting, arm or shoulder touch) or we may touch ourselves (e.g. scratching, nail biting, hair fiddling, chin stroking) or we may touch something else (e.g. pen fiddling, table tapping, foot tapping). Touch can suggest connection or empathy; but it can be dominating or territorial too. Again, touch is culturally sensitive. In Western cultures, handshaking and some form of touch is acceptable and useful, particularly in patients from Latin cultures and many African countries. On the other hand, in some cultures it is not acceptable to touch, particularly between men and women.
- Appearance and environmental clues: how we dress, cut our hair, use make-up or arrange our personal space all gives clues about our interior lives.

40 There is an excellent paper reviewing the evidence about non-verbal communication skills in practice, which is worth reading (Roter *et al.* 2006). Effective non-verbal communication in health practice seems to be associated with a variety of positive patient outcomes. Patients tend to achieve higher levels of functioning, be more satisfied, tend to miss fewer appointments, stick more closely to agreed treatment plans, are more likely to get better, and less likely to sue their doctors. Practitioners who are more skilled in non-verbal communication skills are rated as listening more, being more caring and more sensitive. Particular indicators of good non-verbal communication include more time looking at the patient, more eye contact, more intimate body posture, more head nods and gestures, closer interpersonal distance, amount of time spent gazing at the patient, lower levels of dominance behaviour, higher levels of concern, and more emotionally expressive non-verbal behaviour. Particular indicators of poor non-verbal communication would include distancing behaviours, not smiling, looking away, and frowning. Non-verbal skills are much more highly rated by patients than verbal skills or information giving skills (Roter *et al.* 2006).

41 Image from Prkachin KM. Dissociating spontaneous and deliberate expressions of pain: signal detection analyses. *Pain.* 1992; **51**: 57–65.

42 Other examples would be handshaking (which is considered polite in some societies, and rude in others), a relaxed posture (which may be taken as a compliment or an insult), clothing (which may signify belonging or exclusion), hairstyles (which may signify appropriateness or inappropriateness) and correct speech (which may be considered polite or condescending).

43 We Brits tend to be rather reserved, avoid eye contact, and keep relatively large interpersonal distances. In Uganda, we were amazed by how welcoming, polite and friendly everyone is. It made us feel very embarrassed realising how unwelcome Ugandans must feel when they visit the UK. People always greet each other, even if they have met before that same day. They shake hands, make really good eye

contact, and always ask 'How are you?' (in fact, 'How are you?' is such a widespread form of greeting that small children, even those with no English, would still greet us with a common expression, 'Owaruuu!', which starts low and builds in pitch and volume to end on a prolonged and slightly plaintiff 'uuuuuu!!'). On the other hand, we were sometimes taken aback by how abruptly these conversations would end, often without even a 'goodbye'. At the end of phone conversations, people might simply put the phone down without notice. I don't know if it's true or not, but we were often told that is because welcoming, greeting and taking leave have a much deeper cultural and spiritual significance in Uganda than in England; with welcomes seen as an opportunity to be grateful that we are all still together, but goodbyes avoided in case it suggested that people may not return.

44 *'Wind of drums'* by Chidi Okoye, reproduced by kind permission of the artist. More of Chidi's work can be found on his websites, www.modernartimages.com, www.chidi.com, and www.ArtAfricanArt.com

45 Cues play an important role in how we experience our existence. That is because we experience our existence as a single, integrated whole, not as a series of images or sounds with gaps between. We do this by subconsciously 'filling in' any gaps between sensory signals, and we use 'cues' to gives us clues about how and what to 'fill in'. For example, have you ever wondered how we know what someone would look like from different angles, when we have only seen them from a few? That is because our minds use cues about the size, shape and other signals from the face, and melds these together with other experience of other faces, in order to create the composite whole.

46 Cues can be verbal or non-verbal, very obvious or very subtle. Here are a few examples.

- Verbal cues: these are usually a bit more conscious and might include, for example: repetition of words or phrases (often relating to underling fears or concerns), particularly words like 'serious', 'maybe', 'it's been going on a long time', 'worrying'; emphasising or directing phrases 'you need to understand/know/listen', 'the key/crucial/important point is'; use of strong language or expletives; self-contradiction or self-judgement, e.g. 'It's probably nothing but', or 'I'm sure I am worrying unnecessarily, but'.
- Non-verbal cues: these may be more or less conscious, but are usually fairly obvious, for example: chopping the hand or banging the table to show frustration or anger; exaggerating facial expressions to demonstrate emotional reaction to the verbal message; restlessness of the body, suggestion of agitation of the mind.

47 This is the name given to very fine or subtle behaviours which we may easily miss unless we are trained to pick them up. Originally described by Milton Erikson, they are commonly used by hypnotherapy practitioners but are becoming more widely used in health practice as a way of improving communication, obtaining more information, or of observing how a patient is responding or reacting to discussions. They are the behavioural correlates of confusion, turbulence or dissonance in our minds.

48 Minimal cues might include the following.

- Eye movements: particularly laterally, suggesting patients are accessing either their memories or creative minds.
- Momentary 'trances': where people seem to drift off or freeze temporarily, often because of cognitive dissonance.
- Turbulence in the flow or volume of speech: suggesting repressed emotion of some sort.
- Speech censoring: usually suggesting the patient is hiding something either from themselves or from us (e.g. 'It crossed my mind that . . . but anyway, I was hoping you could help').
- Generalisations: suggesting possible irrational or overvalued ideation (for example: 'I always mess up' or 'I never recover very well').
- Value-laden phrases: for example, 'He's a terrible worrier' or 'She's always the strong one'. These phrases give us a glimpse of the internal 'narratives' and 'dramas' of our patients' lives, and are therefore extremely valuable in helping us work out how best to integrate our suggestions and actions for healing.

49 From Yovel and Kanwisher 2004.

50 People can accurately judge others' emotions based on surprisingly small amounts of behavioural information, often called 'thin slicing'. These thin slices can be very short indeed, usually only a few seconds, and maybe as low as 1 second long. They are therefore perhaps the most efficient form of patient assessment possible. In one thin-slice study participants were exposed to a 5-second audio clip of telephone operators talking to customers and then provided accurate ratings of several different personality traits of the operators. Other studies show that untrained observers can form fairly accurate diagnoses of psychopathology from very thin slices of information, such as voice clips. Of particular interest to practitioners like us, observers could accurately determine the likelihood of doctors being sued simply by listening to short voice clips! (Hecht & LaFrance 1995; Ambady 2002; Fowler *et al*. 2009).

51 Factors such as gender and social adjustment are important (female and better adjusted trainees tend to pick up these skills fastest), but all trainees can be taught to identify and decode non-verbal communication. The core skill to learn is the ability to judge a patient's non-verbal communication (emotional intelligence) and the ability to be able to judge one's own emotional state (emotional self-awareness). The factor that seems to correlate most strongly with both emotional intelligence and self-awareness is greater eye contact (probably because that improves listening skills, picks up more cues, and gives a greater chance of accurately decoding non-verbal communication).

52 When we start training family practitioners who are embarking on their training (residency) programmes in the UK, we spend a lot of time training them in non-verbal communication skills. This is because that, more than anything else, is the factor that decides whether particular consultations run smoothly, quickly, effectively and in a manner that is satisfying both to the patient and doctor. We use videos to do this training, and we can pretty much tell from the first minute of a video how that consultation is going to go. If the trainee doctor starts with a clear and calm mind, manages to establish quick empathic rapport, identifies the patient's overt and covert ideas, concerns and expectations, and accurately identifies and interprets

non-verbal communication, it is rare for the consultation to go wrong. If the trainee doesn't, we know we are in for a much longer, more tortured and possibly ineffective consultation.

53 We can't do much about our height, weight, colour and so on. However, we can influence how we dress, the state of our hair, whether we are shaven or unshaven, the clothes and jewellery we wear, whether we wear uniform and what that looks like, and what accoutrements we carry. Each of these is a symbol of some kind, whether we consciously intend it to be or not. If we are to be effective practitioners, we should consider carefully what these different symbols may mean to the patients that come to see us, and try as far as possible to choose symbols which are integrated with the values, beliefs and approaches of our practice.

54 Transference was originally noted by Freud, and similarly counter-transference soon after. Initially, both were considered to be barriers to therapy. However, as time went on transference became seen as a useful tool. Jung began to explore the possible benefits of counter-transference, using the 'wounded healer' metaphor to explain how the therapist's own problems can be beneficial if they lead to more empathy. However, even then, counter-transference was thought to be something that therapists should become aware of, use for their own healing, but try to avoid with the patient. Gradually, it became clear that counter-transference is nearly as useful as transference as it gives therapists a very clear insight into how the patient is feeling, perhaps even clearer than that of the patients, as well as an opportunity to use transference as a tool to enable patients to mould more healthy self creations. A good book to read is *Transference and Projection* (Grant & Crawley 2002).

55 We are all aware of the fact that our emotions change our expressions, and we can recognise sad, happy or frightened faces in others. However, it appears that the process is two-way, and that changing our facial expression can change the way we feel. So smiling really can make us happy, and frowning can make us feel cross. Kleinke *et al.* (1998) had students view photographs or slides of people with either positive facial expressions (smiling) or negative facial expressions (frowning). Participants in the control group just viewed the photos or slides, participants in the expression group were instructed to mimic the facial expression, and participants in the expression-mirror group matched the expression with the aid of looking in a mirror. As in other studies, facial expressions did affect the participants' mood: mood did not change in the control group who simply viewed the expressions. Participants who matched the positive expressions experienced a positive change in mood (they were in a more positive mood after making positive facial expressions) and participants who matched the negative expressions experienced a negative change in mood. Participants who watched their expressions in a mirror also showed a greater change in mood. It seems that the visual feedback adds to the proprioceptive self-awareness of mood-related facial expression.

56 In this book, we have been talking about the various relationships that we have as sentient beings: the 'me' relationship with ourselves, the 'we' relationship with another person/people, and the 'other' relationship with anything that is not currently in direct relationship with me now. We have also discussed how our existence is both a verb and a noun and the same time. These concepts trace back to Martin

Buber, who was the first to consider existence as a verb, and specifically as an 'encounter'. He suggested that there are two possible encounters 'I–you' and 'I–it' (we have added a third which would be called something like 'I–me' in Buber's language). When we encounter another person we create an infinite, universal and holistic third entity, the 'I–you', within which neither one co-partner is subject or object. When we are not directly encountering other entities, we are still in a form of encounter called the 'I–it' encounter, which is the encounter we have between ourselves and the notion of the other entity that we create in our consciousness. This relationship creates subject (me) and object (it) and enables us to use and experience other objects. However, we can mix these two ideas up, and start to 'objectify' other people, converting our encounter from 'I–you' to 'I–it'. This objectification of other persons enables us to take a scientific, analytic, and material view of existence; but it also creates existential separation between people, with all the conflict and drama this causes. (Buber 2004)

Jacob Levy Moreno first developed the concept of 'encounter' in 1914–16, and it was one of his very early writings (*Invitation to an encounter*) that influenced Buber's ideas in the field of psychology. Buber described all contacts between patient and practitioner as real 'encounters' in which both patient and practitioner create an extemporaneous, unstructured, unplanned, unrehearsed meeting, which is in the here and now. Moreno also developed psychodrama, sociodrama and a whole range of other action/dramatic methods that have since been introduced in a large variety of settings. 'Encounters' are different from empathy, which tends to be one-way (practitioner to patient) and also different from transference (which is a reflection of past experiences), because it is entirely in the here and now. In recognising and acting out these encounters, we get a real and rich experience, wherein for that moment we directly see the world through each other's eyes. From Moreno's work has developed transactional analysis, psychodrama (the acting out of individual existences as a form of therapy) and sociodrama (the acting out of group experiences as a form of group therapy. (With thanks to Zoli Figusch, editor of *From One-to-one Psychodrama to Large Group Socio-psychodrama* (2009) and psychotherapist.)

57 In a similar way to narrative therapy, drama therapy helps patients bring to the surface dramas that they may be acting out in an automated and subconscious way, and thereby try to adapt and change those dramas to make them healthier. Transactional analysis, psychodrama and sociodrama are all useful tools that practitioners can use to explore and express the dramas that underpin and form our lives. In psychodrama and sociodrama, the practitioner helps individual patients or groups of patients to act out particular concerns or issues, and thereby experiment with different plots and outcomes. These practices require time, training and facilities, so are not easily useful to all practitioners, but we can all learn from some of their approaches and techniques.

58 Transactional analysis has a launch point not dissimilar to narrative analysis, in that it suggests every culture, family and individual has a story that explains its/his/her beliefs, values, and aspirations. These stories (or scripts to use dramatic rather than narrative metaphor) are embedded in early childhood and so can contain traces of maladaptive experiences, beliefs and ideas from childhood. These

traces can generate ongoing negative emotions which no longer belong with our adult existence, but which nevertheless get projected onto it. This projection can be self-fulfilling, because if we act them out we will attract other people who wish to act out the reciprocal roles in our drama, often with similar maladaptive issues from their own pasts. By becoming aware of these dramas, we can become aware of the effects of our past experiences and then step free from them.

There is an awful lot more to transactional analysis than we can cover in this book, but please see Eric Berne's (1964) book *Games People Play: the psychology of human relationships*.

59 It's a personal bugbear but don't you find the term 'personality disorder' judgemental, stigmatising and inaccurate? Given that personality is such a relational entity, how can we define when one is 'ordered' or disordered'? As such I have rarely found it to be of any use to the patient. It seems to have utility only to exclude people from services that they would otherwise have had access to.

60 Casey and Tyrer (1990) found that about a third of people attending family practitioners had a personality disorder. Other studies (de Girolamo & Reich 1993; Dowson & Grounds 1995; Moran 1999) have shown between 20% and 40% of patients in mental health clinics and about 50% of mental health inpatients have personality disorder.

61 From Figusch Z, editor. *From One-to-one Psychodrama to Large Group Socio-psychodrama*. Figusch; 2009 (figusch@hotmail.com).

62 Once we have taken a role, the kind of transactions that get acted out vary depending on the roles our fellow actors have taken on. These transactions can be of three different kinds.

- Reciprocal: when we address the 'correct' role that the other is in (e.g. adult to child, victim to persecutor).
- Crossed: when we address a role that the other is not in (e.g. adult to child when the partner wishes to play the adult).
- Covert: when one person plays two different roles at once, expressing one overtly and the other covertly (e.g. when a patient demands help, in an overt parent role, but rejects or sabotages whatever help is offered, in a covert child role).

63 If we are under pressure from other people to come out of the drama (because they won't play their roles, or question ours), we often use our psychological defences to stay within our drama. For example, we can 'redefine' what other people are saying or doing (e.g. so an apparently kind action towards us when we are in the victim mode is reinterpreted as manipulative abuse). Alternatively, we can discount that kindness so that it does not challenge our view of the other as persecutor. Discounting can be 'acted out' by ignoring, becoming passive, becoming angry, becoming unsettled or agitated or even violent.

64 This poem was written by Jessica Napoli under the pseudonym 'Blair Witch'. She wrote it partly for cathartic reasons and therapeutic relief, but also hoping it would help others as well. She stipulates that she does not want her poem to be used in any way that will make people suffering from BPD look 'crazy'. I hope that readers will see that my intention is the opposite: to try to demonstrate the health practitioners that people with BPD and other personality disorders are just the same as anyone

else, but they have the added burden of living and coping with often profound difficulties in their lives. From www.gotpoetry.com

65 'Do not go gentle into that good night', by Dylan Thomas, from *The Poems of Dylan Thomas*, revised edition. New York: New Directions; 2003. Reprinted with kind permission of New Directions Books.

66 'The House that Fear Built: Warsaw, 1943', by Jane Flanders from *Timepiece*, published by the University of Pittsburgh Press (1988) and reprinted by kind permission of the Estate of Jane Flanders and the University of Pittsburgh Press.

67 Play allows children to practise for later life, but there seems to be much more to it than that. Freud regarded play as cathartic: helping children release negative feelings caused by traumatic events and substitute them with more positive ones, so that it could help children come to understand painful situations and find ways to substitute pleasurable feelings for unpleasant ones; so that it would help children to master their covert thoughts and overt actions; and lastly so that it would help them to learn to interpret their experiences. Certainly, as children begin to realise their own vulnerability in their enormous world, play can help children reduce this sense of vulnerability. Perhaps that is why children like to play with miniature toys, reducing the overwhelming world of adults to a manageable size.

Psychoanalytic theorists, such as Erik Erikson, suggested that play mirrors and supports a child's psychological and social development. In the first year of life, children use their sensory and motor skills to explore their own bodies. In the second year, they progress to manipulating objects in the environment. These play activities can help children develop their self-esteem and sense of empowerment by allowing them mastery of objects. Gradually, as they play, children go beyond control of objects to mastery of social interactions with their peers.

Piaget, a cognitive theorist, considered play to be a major tool for facilitating children's mental development and as a means of facilitating learning by exposing 'a child to new experiences and new possibilities of physical and mental activities for dealing with the world'. Piaget believed that people change their ways of thinking and behaving in order to adapt to their environments and that such adaptation is important for physical survival and psychological/intellectual growth. In Piaget's stage theory, the changes in play through each stage parallel different levels of cognitive and emotional development. They enable children to practise thoughts and behaviours that are acceptable to society so that they can act appropriately in different situations. Different kinds of play require different levels of cognitive sophistication, and that is why each different type of play is found at a specific stage of cognitive development.

Vygotsky, a sociocultural theorist, believed that play serves as a tool of the mind to help children master their behaviours. This theory suggests that the function of play is to help children develop self-regulation, expand the separation between their thought and actions, and develop the skills needed to obtain a higher cognitive functioning. For example, when a child builds a car from wire or from blocks, he is learning to separate out the thought or image of the car (the toy) from the actual car he is trying to conceptualise or represent. This separation between actual and symbolic worlds, between thought and action, prepares children to develop abstract thinking. Thinking and acting are no longer simultaneous; behaviours are no longer driven by objects, but rather by children's symbolic thought. Play allows children to try out different thoughts and behaviours, mapping these to the real world, and therefore children become capable of using high-level mental functions (i.e. abstract thinking) to manipulate and monitor thoughts and ideas without direct and immediate reference to the real world. Therefore, play is an important educational strategy for facilitating children's development in cognitive, social/emotional, motor, and language areas.

Caplan and Caplan, picking up Freud's themes, suggest that children deliberately create a make-believe play world for themselves in which they can experience a sense of freedom, control and mastery. In this world they can manipulate reality and feel empowered. As they master their world, play helps children develop new competencies that lead to enhanced confidence and the resiliency they will need to face future challenges. More recent theories have emphasised that the process is not one way. In other words, it is not simply that play develops as the brain develops. It works the other way around as well. Play helps the brain to develop. A child's development is critically mediated by appropriate, affective relationships with loving and consistent caregivers as they relate to children through play. Without play, children's brains and capacities will not develop healthily. This is of particular importance where children are already suffering with physical illnesses which themselves inhibit development.

Play might be cathartic (Freud), it can mirror and supports a child's psychological and social development contributing to the full emotional development of the child (Erikson), change a child's way of thinking and behaving in order to adapt to their environments (Piaget), serve as a tool of the mind to help children master their behaviours (Vygotsky), experience a sense of freedom, control, and mastery. (Caplan & Caplan 1973; Pepler 1982).

68 There are different ways of classifying play, for example:

- Attunement play: when an infant makes eye contact with her mother, each experiences a spontaneous surge of emotion (joy). The baby responds with a radiant smile, the mother with her own smile and rhythmic vocalisations (baby talk).

- Motor/physical play: motor play provides critical opportunities for children to develop both individual gross and fine muscle strength and overall integration of muscles, nerves and brain functions. Learning about self-movement structures an individual's knowledge of the world – it is a way of knowing, and we actually, through movement and play, think in motion. For example, the play-driven movement of leaping upward is a lesson about gravity as well as one's body.

- Social play: by interacting with others in play settings, children learn social rules such as give and take, reciprocity, cooperation and sharing. Through a range of interactions with children at different social stages, children also learn to use moral reasoning to develop a mature sense of values.

- Play and belonging: the urge to play with others, in addition to being fun, is often driven by the desire to be accepted, to belong. This starts with 'parallel' play but later, as development proceeds, friendships begin to develop and empathy for others forms. Group loyalty and affection ensues, and with it the rudiments of a

ment to create things. This type of play occurs when children build towers and
cities with blocks, play in the sand, construct contraptions on the woodworking
bench, and draw pictures with chalk on the sidewalk. Constructive play allows
children to experiment with objects; find out combinations that work and don't
work; and learn basic knowledge about stacking, building, drawing, making
music and constructing. Along with other special patterns of play, the curiosity
about and playing with 'objects' is a pervasive innately fun pattern of play, and
creates its own 'states' of playfulness. Early on, toys take on highly personalised
characteristics, and as skills in manipulating objects (i.e. banging on pans, skipping rocks, etc.) develop, the richer become the circuits in the brain. Hands
playing with all types of objects help brains develop beyond strictly manipulative
skills, with play as the driver of this development. The correlation of effective
adult problem solving and earlier encouragement of and facility in manipulating
objects has been established. It also gives children a sense of accomplishment
and empowers them with control of their environment. Children who are comfortable manipulating objects and materials also become good at manipulating
words, ideas and concepts.

- Fantasy play: children learn to abstract, to try out new roles and possible
situations, and to experiment with language and emotions with fantasy play.
In addition, children develop flexible thinking; learn to create beyond the here
and now; stretch their imaginations; use new words and word combinations in
a risk-free environment; and use numbers and words to express ideas, concepts,
dreams and histories.

- Games with rules: developmentally, most children progress from an egocentric
view of the world to an understanding of the importance of social contracts and
rules. Part of this development occurs as they learn that games like Follow the
Leader, Red Rover, Simon Says, soccer and other team sports cannot function
without everyone adhering to the same set of rules. The 'games with rules' concept

162

teaches children a critically important concept – the game of life has rules (laws) that we all must follow to function productively.

69 Play encourages physical development (e.g. running, climbing, throwing, lifting and carrying), releases energy, provides challenges, allows the child to repeat and practise important skills, encourages emotional development, builds self-esteem, aids expression and understanding of emotions, acts out inner fears and anxieties, enables them to take risks and to make decisions, and uses imagination. It helps a child look at things from new perspectives, encourages social skills such as sharing, negotiating and resolving conflicts, teaches self-advocacy skills, develops considera- tion and empathy, and play helps the child try out different social roles, become more aware of identity, and forget worries and concerns; it encourages thinking and language development, intellectual flexibility, helps them adjust to new challenges, learn readiness, learn behaviours and problem-solving skills, understand concepts (e.g. up and down, hard and soft, big and small), learn to sort and classify, explore and solve problems and improve ability to concentrate. Finally, play also gives a valuable opportunity to have fun and experience pure delight and happiness!

70 Child development is not fixed but context dependent. A child with more stimula- tion in a particular area is likely to develop faster down that 'developmental line' than others. This is why children who have more experience of illness and death often have advanced understanding in that area. Therefore, we should not pre-judge a child's understanding on the basis of developmental charts. Each child needs to be assessed and understood in their own right. Children can develop at different rates down different developmental lines: one child might develop quickly with physical and language skills, but less quickly with intellectual skills. A child might be quite 'bright' cognitively, but be limited in social or moral skills. Therefore we should not assume that an 'advanced' child is advanced in all areas; or that a 'slow' child is slow in all areas.

71 Kandel, Schwartz & Jessell (2000). Very real chemical and physical changes take place in the brain during these critical learning periods. This is a time when a child will learn a new skill (such as language or reading) with very little effort. During this period the child's visual, mental and motor systems are ready to be used and, if triggered by the environment, they will be used together most effectively for the learning of the skill or task. In other words, the young child's brain is still 'plastic'. It can still grow, adapt and make new neuronal connections in response to stimuli. On the other hand, in the absence of relevant stimulation, parts of the brain become inactive, shrink down and eventually stop functioning altogether. Eyesight, motion, balance, hearing, speech, and even the ability to form close and loving relationships can be permanently lost if a child is not properly stimulated in the crucial first few years.

72 BC Mills in the book *The Child under Six* (Hymes 1994).

73 For example:
- Freud's psychosexual stage theory; the oral, anal, phallic, latent and genital stages.
- Piaget's theory of cognitive development: looking at how children represent and reason about the world.

- Erikson's stages of psychosocial development: explaining how children recognise, confront and have to overcome new challenges at different stages of their lives.
- Fowler's stages of faith theory: suggesting that we go through different stages of spiritual development and understanding.
- Kohlberg's stages of moral development from pre-conventional (self-interested obedience and conformity) to conventional (interpersonal understanding and agreement about order and conformity) and post-conventional (exploration of social contracts and universal moral principles).
- Maslow's hierarchy of needs.
- Beck and Cowan's 'Spiral Dynamics': suggesting that we continuously redefine and adapt to changing conditions of our lives, by creating and expressing ever more complex and relational conceptual models of our existence. Each stage revisits (hence circles back) but also includes and transcends (hence builds upon) previous models. The continuous circling but developing is represented as a spiral rather than a circle, as it has a forward trajectory as well as a circular nature.

74 It may be that you have very little space in which to operate. However, in case you do, we have suggested below some ideas for how you might want to set up an area for the children in your care. In general terms it is good to have:
- a cognitive (thinking) area – for children to think and learn
- a book area – for children to read and be read to
- a fantasy area – for dressing up and puppet plays
- a creative area – for painting, drawing, creative play and crafts
- an outdoor area – for energetic play
- a sleeping area – for sleep and rest.

75 Freud considered rituals (particularly religious rituals) to be remnants of childish fantasy, but ritual can also be seen as crucial for humans to make and share sense of the world around them. Like other creative activities, they use symbols and actions to explore things that logic and words cannot. Durkheim, on the other hand, suggested that rituals are key social interactions that are at the heart of all family, cultural and social identity, which create group emotions, identities and meaning; act as a basis for beliefs and morality; and link these to symbolic entities so creating foundations upon which cultures and societies can found and develop themselves. The cycle of interaction → emotions → symbols → interaction forms patterns of interaction over time and place and therefore acts as a crucial structural force that organises groups, societies and cultures. (Durkheim 2001)

76 Rituals help us to recognise and become part of a familial, cultural and social identity and provide us with opportunities for expression of, and inclusion within, those identities. By taking part in, and then discussing, rituals, we tell and retell ourselves narratives which give our life structure and meaning. When these narratives are linked with many previous generations through the knowledge that our ancestors carried out the same rituals in the same way, they give us a direct link to, and union with, our past and our roots, as well as identity in the present.

77 Originally described by Albert Bandura, self-efficacy is basically our belief in our ability to succeed. Bandura studied how we learn and develop by observing and testing our learning in social contexts. If we have high self-efficacy we will believe

we can take on and succeed in new things, we develop deeper interests, and form stronger commitments. If we don't have a strong self-efficacy we may avoid new challenges, lose heart more easily and tend to focus on our failings rather than successes. Self-efficacy seems to start to form in early childhood but continues throughout life; and always develops in response to acquisition of new skills, experiences, and understandings. Bandura suggested there are four sources of self-efficacy: mastery experiences (when we succeed at something); social modelling (watching others succeed at something); social persuasion (when others encourage us we can do something) and psychological response (where emotions like anxiety and heightened awareness either impede or enhance our chances of success). (Bandura 1977)

78 *Evidence: Helping people help themselves. A review of the evidence considering whether it is worthwhile to support self-management*. Health Foundation, May 2011. Reprinted with kind permission of the Health Foundation.

79 In family practice, non-adherence to treatment recommendations is 20% to 40% for acute illness, 30% to 60% for chronic illness, and 80% for prevention. These result in ineffective treatment and poor outcomes. Although it was originally developed for the treatment of addictions, motivational interviewing has been widely adapted to facilitate change across a range of patient health behaviours, including those related to the management and prevention of chronic diseases. Motivational interviewing is well suited for use in many healthcare settings because it can be applied in very brief (10-to-15-minute) patient encounters. (Levensky, Forcehimes & Beitz 2007)

80 'Bad Habits' by Dwayne Carter, reprinted with kind permission of the artist and also of J R Compton, Editor/Publisher off the Dallas Arts Revue at http:DallasArtsRevue.com (where more of Dwayne's work, and that of other artists, can be seen.

81 Smoking, excessive alcohol consumption, lack of exercise and an unhealthy diet cause premature morbidity and mortality. Brief interventions in healthcare consultations can be effective in changing single health behaviours. Simply telling a patient to stop smoking increases their chances of success, although only from 4% to 8% per attempt. (NICE 2006)

82 Evidence for motivational interviewing is emerging, although not always consistently supportive. Studies showing particular benefits include treatment for drug and alcohol abuse and smoking, but also for treatment adherence, HIV risk reduction, diet and exercise, and health safety practices. An important finding is that it is the quality of the commitment to change (rather than the frequency of discussion about change) that is most important, which suggests practitioners need to focus closely on what patients are communicating, verbally and non-verbally, about patients' values, assumptions, fears and hopes in order to ensure interventions are most fruitful and not wasted. Several studies have also found that motivational interviewing has promising effects when compared with standard approaches, such as patient education, risk reduction interventions, nonspecific counselling, and treatment contracts. (McCambridge 2004; Grimshaw 2006; Soria, Legido & Escolano 2006).

83 The Transtheoretical Model (Prochaska 1994) or Stages of Change Model suggests that we change by moving through several stages, as follows.

- Precontemplation: where we are unaware that there is anything we need to change.
- Contemplation: where we are aware we may need to change, but have not done anything about it yet.
- Preparation: where we start making small movements in the direction of change, to prepare ourselves.
- Action: where we try to make the change.
- Maintenance: where we have made the change and work hard to avoid going backwards.
- Termination: where the change is complete and we have no desire to return to the pre-changed state.

84 This poem is in the public domain.

85 Although this may seem quite a straightforward question, it turns out to be a bit more complicated than we might think. We have seen how things like values, knowledge and effectiveness are self-referential, relational, leaky and blurry concepts. As decisions are choices based upon values, knowledge and predicted effectiveness, it is not so surprising to discover that decisions are also relational, leaky and blurry concepts too.

86 Economists have a number of theories about how we make decisions and value the outcomes. These include the following.

- Rational decision making: where we use consistent, logical reasoning. However, it appears we are often not rational or don't have sufficient grasp of logic, maths or probability to make judgements.
- Expected value theory: where we calculate the potential value of each option and pick the option with the highest expected value. However, value is contextual and subjective (e.g. $1 to a rich man is worth much less than $1 to a poor man).
- Expected utility: where we decide how useful an outcome might be for us. However, this may lead to irrational decisions (e.g. in the lottery the utility value of the cost of the ticket is low, but the utility value of the prize may be very high).
- Certainty bias: people often prefer the certain rather than the beneficial, but unfortunately nothing in life is that certain.
- Gains and losses bias: people are more likely to avoid risks that might lead to losses than they are to take risks that might lead to gains, which (along with the certainty bias) makes us quite conservative in decision making.
- Framing bias: the way we frame the question influences the answer, e.g. a relative risk reduction of 50% sounds much better than an absolute risk reduction of 1% (from 2%).
- Context effects: the context of a decision heavily influences the decision (so I may be happy to buy a new iPhone when I am feeling happy, but less so when I am feeling down – although it may be the other way round).
- Uncertain probabilities: we can use probability to make value. Bookies do this very well, punters less so, which is why they are rich and we are not.
- Complexity: where decisions have so many variables we can't even work out the probability let alone the answer.

87 Social cognitive theory looks at the way we perceive and judge, and what the

influences on our perceptions and judgements may be. These together make up 'social knowledge', which has an effect on what and how we decide. In the health sphere, social theory suggests that a number of non-medical factors influence decision making:

- characteristics of the patient: age, gender, socioeconomic status, race/ethnicity, language and physical appearance
- the organisational setting
- the signs and symptoms of disease
- the characteristics of the doctor: including specialty, level of training, clinical experience, age, gender and race/ethnicity
- characteristics of the practice: including location, organisation of practice, form of compensation, performance expectations, and incentives
- natural tendencies to stereotype
- prejudice and discrimination.

McKinlay summarises, *'Medical decision making can be as much a function of who the patient is as much as what the patient has.'* Recent literature supports this and challenges the prescriptive theory of decision making. For instance, there are significant geographic variations in procedure utilisation for the same clinical condition across the country (Betancourt & Ananeh-Firempong 2004).

88 We may like to think we are objective, but it appears that we treat decisions about our own health quite differently to the way we treat decisions about our patients' health (we tend to choose the treatment with the greatest chance of survival for our patients, but with the lowest risk of side effects for ourselves). This may be because we let our emotions and values play more of a role when thinking about our own health. (Ubel, Angott & Zikmund-Fischer 2011).

89 The way statistics are described makes a difference to how they are interpreted and applied. So a relative risk reduction of 50% sounds much better than an absolute risk reduction of 1% (from 2%), even though it's the same thing.

90 The UK Department of Health 'Shared Decision Making' website also shows that in all cases except hysterectomy and prostatectomy, shared decision making reduces the numbers choosing surgery (which of course is wonderful news to the accountants, if not for the surgeons). (Lewin *et al.* 2001).

91 *Cochrane review.* Two Cochrane reviews have shown that, where 'shared decision making' has been tried out, it seems there are several beneficial effects, for example reductions in unnecessary treatments, improved concordance with care, better quality of care, increased satisfaction (for both patients and medical staff), improved self-esteem for patients, improving clinical safety, reduction in unwarranted practice variation, and reduced litigation costs. They also suggest that shared decision making produces better quality of care, increased satisfaction (for both patients and medical staff), and improved self-esteem for patients. Barriers to implementation in practice include practitioners' attitudes and skills, time available, personal preferences, experiences, and relationships; and structural constraints (class, education, ethnicity and culture). They will also vary over time as people are more exposed or familiar with involvement in decision making and to vary from one situation or context to another for an individual patient. People tend to show potentially

contradictory or ambivalent stands in relation to assuming responsibility for their health and healthcare at different times and in different situations.

Another Cochrane review showed that the most effective interventions to promote shared decision making were practitioner educational meetings, giving practitioners feedback about their shared decision making skills, giving practitioners learning materials, and using patient decision aids. (Légaré *et al.* 2011).

92 Research shows that some patients wish to share decision making with practitioners, but others don't. This may be an issue if the practitioner's recommendations are coercive, because the practitioner's recommendations are powerful influences on the patient's decisions. Indeed, physician recommendations have been shown to have a strong influence on patients' decisions. On the other hand, patients may (and do) make choices that are apparently not in their best interests, particularly when they are very unwell, have reduced capacity or are anxious. In such situations, practitioners can be more 'objective', and so less susceptible to cognitive biases than patients. When people make decisions for others, they tend to hone in on the most important aspect of the decision and are less swayed by extraneous factors that could bias the decision. (Deber 1996; Sandman & Munthe 2010; Ubel, Angott & Zikmund-Fischer 2011)

93 'Table Talk' by Juliana Burrell, reproduced with kind permission of the artist, whose work can be seen at www.julianaburrell.com

94 The main barriers to shared decision making (Sandman & Munthe 2010) in practice seem to be the following.

- Practitioners: may be put off by the apparent challenge to our autonomy, may not recognise preference sensitive decisions, or find that the evidence is difficult to extract, interpret or communicate.
- Practice: there are logistical challenges including lack of time and lack of reimbursement or incentivisation compared to other activities.
- Patients: may not want to participate, may vary in their role preference, and may not be literate or numerate or able to manipulate probabilities.

The things that seem to support shared decision making the most include:
- education and training of practitioners (about how to carry out shared decision making)
- patient feedback to practitioners about their shared decision-making skills
- provision of learning materials for patients and practitioners
- formal patient decision aids.

95 The evidence suggests (Légaré *et al.* 2010) that decisions that should take the highest priority for shared decision making include the following.

- Where there is more than one possible approach.
- Where the interventions may be risky.
- Where there are significant cultural or subcultural differences between patient and practitioner.
- Where the treatment will involve a lot of patient input.
- Where the treatment requires close concordance.
- Where the treatment requires significant lifestyle changes.

96 Patient decision aids (PDA) are tools designed to help patients make difficult

treatment or screening decisions when there is no clinical evidence in favour of one single best option. They aim to increase patients' awareness of the expected risks, benefits and likely outcomes, empowering them to make informed choices about their care. Some very useful examples of PDAs are available on the UK 'NHS Direct' website (www.nhsdirect.nhs.uk/DecisionAids).

97 Issues that affect how successful shared decision making might be include whether the causes can be overcome, how sick the patient will be, what the outlook is, previous good or bad experiences, the level of social support, the viability of the treatment options, the likelihood of success or failure, the patient's ability to tolerate risk and manage failure, any resources that exist or may be needed, and the people that need to be involved. Most importantly, time. Much of this takes time, and usually more time than a typical practitioner has in typical practice. And it's not just a question of time. There is usually a limit to what patient (and practitioner) can deal with in one sitting. For both these reasons, much of this process has to be broken into chunks and managed over a time line.

98 'What the doctor said' by Raymond Carver, from *A New Path to the Waterfall* by Raymond Carver, published 13 January 1994 by Atlantic Monthly Press (first published 1989). Reprinted with kind permission of Atlantic Monthly Press.

99 Even less frequently studied is emotional self-awareness, although this is recognised as an attribute of the reflective practitioner, with some authors asserting that awareness of one's own feelings is a prerequisite for insights into the feelings of others and an indication of empathic ability.

Bibliography

Abbasi K. Doctors: automatons, technicians, or knowledge brokers? *JRSM*. 2007; **100**(1): 1. Print.

Aked J, Marks N, Cordon C, Thompson S. Five ways to well-being. *Foresight Project on Mental Capital and Wellbeing*. New Economics Foundation; 2008. Web. Available at: www.neweconomics.org/publications/five-ways-well-being-evidence

Alladin A, Alibhai A. Cognitive hypnotherapy for depression: an empirical investigation. *IJCEH*. 2007; **55**(2): 147–66. Print.

Allen RP. *Scripts and Strategies in Hypnotherapy: the complete works*. Carmarthen: Crown House Publishing; 2004. Print.

Ambady N. Surgeons' tone of voice: a clue to malpractice history. *Surgery*. 2002; **132**(1): 5–9. Print.

Amery J. *Children's Palliative Care in Africa*. Oxford: Oxford University Press; 2009. Print.

Anielski M. *The Economics of Happiness: building genuine wealth*. Gabriola, BC: New Society; 2007. Print.

Armstrong D. Space and time in British general practice. *Soc Sci Med*. 1985; **20**(7): 659–66. Print.

Arnetz BB, Horte LG. Suicide patterns among physicians related to other academics as well as to the general populations: results from a national long-term prospective study and a retrospective study. *Acta Psychiatr Scand*. 1987; **75**(2): 139–43. Print.

Balint M. *The Doctor, His Patient, and the Illness*. New York: International Universities; 1957. Print.

Bandura A. Self-efficacy: toward a unifying theory of behavioral change. *Psychol Rev*. 1977; **84**(2): 191–215. Print.

Barsky AJ. Hidden reasons some patients visit doctors. *Ann Intern Med*. 1981; **94**: 492–8. Print.

Beating the Blues®. Web. Available at: www.beatingtheblues.co.uk (accessed 28 October 2011).

Beck DE, Cowan CC. *Spiral Dynamics*. Oxford: Blackwell; 2006. Print.

Beckman HB, Frankel RM. The effect of physician behavior on the collection of data. *Ann Intern Med*. 1984; **101**: 692–6. Print.

Beevers CG, Miller IW. Perfectionism, cognitive bias, and hopelessness as prospective predictors of suicidal ideation. *Suicide and Life-Threatening Behavior*. 2004; **34**(2): 126–37. Print.

Bench M. Open Door Coaching. Web. Available at: www.opendoorcoaching.com. (accessed 17 October 2011). Copyright © 2003 Marcia Bench and Career Coach Institute; reprinted with permission.

Berne E. *Games People Play: the psychology of human relationships*. New York: Grove; 1964. Print.

Betancourt JR, Ananeh-Firempong O. Not me! Doctors, decisions, and disparities in health care: how do we really make decisions? *Cardiovasc Rev Rep*. 2004; **25**(3): n.p. Print.

Better Health. Web. Available at: http://getbetterhealth.com (accessed 17 October 2011).

Black Dog Institute. *Depression*. Black Dog Institute. Web. Available at: www.black doginstitute.org.au (accessed 23 November 2011).

Blanck PD, Buck R, Rosenthal R. *Nonverbal Communication in the Clinical Context*. University Park: Pennsylvania State University Press; 1986. Print.

Blenkiron P. *Stories and Analogies in Cognitive Behavioural Therapy*. Oxford: Wiley Blackwell; 2010. Print.

Block N. How many concepts of consciousness? *Behavioral and Brain Sciences*. 1995; **18**(2):272–8. Print.

BMJ. How much do we know? Clinical Evidence. BMJ. Web. Available at: http://clinical evidence.bmj.com/ceweb/about/knowledge.jsp (accessed 17 October 2011)

Bohm D. *Wholeness and the Implicate Order*. London: Routledge & Kegan Paul; 1981. Print.

Bradford VTS. Trainers' Toolkit. Home. Web. Available at: www.bradfordvts.co.uk (accessed 12 November 2011).

Brantley J. *Calming Your Anxious Mind: how mindfulness and compassion can free you from anxiety, fear, and panic*. Oakland, CA: New Harbinger Publications; 2007. Print.

British Association for Behavioural & Cognitive Psychotherapies. Home Page. Web. Available at: www.babcp.com (accessed 28 October 2011).

British Medical Association. *Doctors' Health*. 8 May 2007. Web. Available at: www.bma. org.uk/doctors_health/doctorshealth.jsp?page=2 (accessed 28 October 2011).

British Medical Association. *Quality and Outcomes Framework, February 2010*. Web. Available at: www.bma.org.uk/employmentandcontracts/independent_contractors/ quality_outcomes_framework/qualityframework10.jsp (accessed 28 October 2011).

Brown D. Evidence-based hypnotherapy for asthma: a critical review. *IJCEH*. 2007; **55**(2): 220–49. Print.

Bruton HJ. Book review: nations and households in economic growth: essays in honor of Moses Abramovitz (Paul A. David, Melvin W. Reder). *Economic Development and Cultural Change*. 1979; **27**(4): 801. Print.

Bstan-'dzin-rgya-mtsho, Hopkins J. *Becoming Enlightened*. New York: Atria; 2009. Print.

Buber M. *I and Thou*. New York: Continuum; 2004. Print.

Buchbinder SB, Wilson M, Melick CF. Estimates of costs of primary care physician turnover. *Am J Managed Care*. 1999; **5**(11): 1431. Print.

Businessballs. *Job Satisfaction Inventory*. Businessballs Free Online Learning for Careers, Work, Management, Business Training and Education. Web. Available at: http:// businessballs.com (accessed 27 October 2011).

Businessballs. Web. Available at: http://businessballs.com (accessed 24 October 2011).

Byrne PS, Long BEL. *Doctors Talking to Patients*. London: HMSO; 1978. Print.

Campbell DT. Blind variation and selective retention in creative thought as in other knowledge processes. *Psychol Rev.* 1960; **67**: 380–400. Print.

Campling P, Haigh R. *Therapeutic Communities: past, present, and future.* London: Jessica Kingsley; 1999. Print.

Campo R. What the body told. *The World in Us: lesbian and gay poetry of the next wave.* New York: Griffin; 2001. N.p. Print.

Caplan F, Caplan T. *The Power of Play.* New York: Doubleday; 1973. Print.

Carroll L, Green RL. *Alice's Adventures in Wonderland; and, through the looking-glass and what Alice found there.* London: Oxford University Press; 1971. Print.

Casey PR, Tyrer P. Personality disorder and psychiatric illness in general practice. *Br J Psychiatry.* 1990; **156**(2): 261–5. Print.

Chomsky N. A minimalist program for linguistic theory. *The View from the Building: essays in honor of Sylvain Bromberger.* Cambridge: MIT; 1993. N.p. Print.

Cole SA, Bird J. *The Medical Interview: the three-function approach.* St. Louis: Mosby; 2000. Print.

Committee on the Use of Complementary and Alternative Medicine by the American Public. *Complementary and Alternative Medicine in the United States.* Washington, DC: National Academies; 2005. Print.

Covey, S. *The 7 Habits Of Highly Effective People.* Free Press; Revised edition 2004.

Cozens J. Doctors, their wellbeing and stress. *BMJ.* 2003; **326**: 670–1. Print.

Csikszentmihalyi M. *Finding Flow: the psychology of engagement with everyday life.* New York: Basic; 1997. Print.

Dalai Lama. *Becoming Enlightened.* London: Rider; 2010. Print.

Dalai Lama, Cutler HC. *The Art of Happiness: a handbook for living.* Audiobook CD. New York: Simon & Schuster Audio; 1998.

Dalai Lama, Hopkins J. *Becoming Enlightened.* New York: Atria; 2009. Print.

Damgaard-Mørch NL, Nielsen LJ, Uldwall SW. [Knowledge and perceptions of complementary and alternative medicine among medical students in Copenhagen]. [Article in Danish] Ugeskr Laeger. 2008; **170**(48): 3941–5. Available in translation at: www. vifab.dk/uk/statistics/medical+students+and+alternative+medicine?

Davison S. Principles of managing patients with personality disorder. *Adv Psychiatr Treat.* 2002; **8**: 1–9. Print.

Deber RB. What role do patients wish to play in treatment decision making? *Arch Intern Med.* 1996; **156**: 1414–20. Print.

de Girolamo G, Reich JH. *Epidemiology of Mental Disorders and Psychosocial Problems: personality disorders.* Geneva: World Health Organization; 1993. Print.

DeLongis A, Folkman S, Lazarus RS. The impact of daily stress on health and mood: psychological and social resources as mediators. *J Pers Soc Psychol.* 1988; **54**(3): 486–95. Print.

Dennett DC. *Consciousness Explained.* London: Penguin; 1993. Print.

Deveugele M, Derese A, van den Brink-Muinen A, *et al.* Consultation length in general practice: cross sectional study in six European countries. *BMJ.* 2002; **325**(7362): 472. Print.

Dewey J. *How We Think.* Boston: D.C. Heath & Co; 1910. Print.

Dickinson E, Franklin RW. *The Poems of Emily Dickinson*. Cambridge, MA: Belknap of Harvard University Press; 1998. Print.

Digman JM. Personality structure: emergence of the five-factor model. *Annu Rev Psychology.* 1990; **41**(1): 417–40. Print.

DiMatteo M, Robin CD, Sherbourne RD, *et al*. Physicians' characteristics influence patients' adherence to medical treatment: results from the Medical Outcomes Study. *Health Psychol.* 1993; **12**(2): 93–102. Print.

DOH. *Improving Access to Psychological Therapies (IAPT) Programme: computerised Cognitive Behavioural Therapy (cCBT) implementation guidance.* Department of Health, UK; March 2007. Web. Available at: www.dh.gov.uk/en/Publicationsand statistics/Publications/PublicationsPolicyAndGuidance/DH_073470

DOH. *Delivering Care, Improving Outcomes for Patients.* Quality and Outcomes Framework; 8 February 2010.

DOH. *Mental Health and Ill Health in Doctors.* London: Crown Publishing; 2008. Department of Health. Web. Available at: www.dh.gov.uk/en/Publicationsandstatistics/ Publications/PublicationsPolicyAndGuidance/DH_083066.

DOH. *Mental Health Policy Implementation Guide: adult acute inpatient care provision.* Department of Health (UK); 2002. Web. Available at: www.positive-options.com/ news/downloads/DoH_-_Adult_Acute_In-patient_Care_Provision_-_2002.pdf.

DOH. *The GP Patient Survey: general information.* The GP Patient Survey. UK Department of Health; 2010. Web. Available at: www.gp-patient.co.uk/info

Doran T. Effect of financial incentives on incentivised and non-incentivised clinical activities: longitudinal analysis of data from the UK Quality and Outcomes Framework. *BMJ.* 2011; **342**: 590–8. Print.

Dowson JH, Grounds A. *Personality Disorders: recognition and clinical management.* Cambridge: Cambridge University Press; 1995. Print.

Dunnette MD, Hough LM, Triandis HC. *Handbook of Industrial and Organizational Psychology.* Palo Alto, CA: Consulting Psychologists; 1990. Print.

Durkheim É, Cladis CS. *The Elementary Forms of Religious Life.* Oxford: Oxford University Press; 2001. Print.

Durojave OC. Health screening: is it always worth doing? *The Internet Journal of Epidemiology.* 2009; **7**(1): n.p. Print.

Easterlin RA. Does economic growth improve the human lot? Some empirical evidence. In: David PA, Reder MW, editors. *Nations and Households in Economic Growth: essays in honor of Moses Abramovitz.* New York: Academic Press; 1974. Print.

Edelman GM, Mountcastle VB. *The Mindful Brain: cortical organization and the group-selective theory of higher brain function.* Cambridge: MIT; 1978. Print.

Edelman GM, Tononi G. *A Universe of Consciousness: how matter becomes imagination.* New York, NY: Basic; 2000. Print.

Ely JW, Osheroff JA, Ebell M. Analysis of questions asked by family doctors regarding patient care. *BMJ.* 1997; **319**: 358–61. Print.

Epstein RM. Mindful practice. *JAMA.* 1999; **292**(9): 833. Print.

Eraut M. Non-formal learning and tacit knowledge in professional work. *Br J Educ Psychol.* 2000; **70**(1): 113–36. Print.

Erickson HC, Tomlin EM, Price Swain MA. *Modeling and Role Modeling: a theory and paradigm for nursing*. Englewood Cliffs, NJ: Prentice-Hall; 1983. Print.

Ericsson KA. *The Cambridge Handbook of Expertise and Expert Performance*. Cambridge: Cambridge University Press; 2006. Print.

Ernst E. Obstacles to research in complementary and alternative medicine. *Med J Aust.* 2003; **179**(6): 279–80. Print.

Evans R. Releasing time to care: Productive Ward, survey results. *Nurs Times.* 2007; **10**(Suppl. 16): S6–9.

Eve R. *PUNs and DENs: discovering learning needs in general practice*. Oxford: Radcliffe Medical Press; 2003. Print.

Everett DL. *Don't Sleep, There Are Snakes: life and language in the Amazonian jungle*. New York: Pantheon; 2008. Print.

FearFighter. Panic & Phobia Treatment. CCBT Limited Healthcare online. Web. Available at: www.fearfighter.com

Festinger L. *A Theory of Cognitive Dissonance*. California: Stanford University Press; 1957. Print.

Figusch Z, editor. *From One-to-one Psychodrama to Large Group Socio-psychodrama: more writings from the arena of Brazilian psychodrama*. Figusch; 2009. Print.

Finke RA, Ward TB, Smith SM. *Creative Cognition: theory, research, and applications*. Cambridge, MA: MIT; 1996. Print.

Firth-Cozens J. Doctors, their wellbeing, and their stress. *BMJ.* 2003; **326**: 670–1. Print.

Flett G. York researcher finds that perfectionism can lead to imperfect health. *York's Daily Bulletin*. Toronto, Canada: York University; June 2004. Print.

Flood GD. *An Introduction to Hinduism*. New York, NY: Cambridge University Press; 1996. Print.

Flynn JR. *What Is Intelligence: beyond the Flynn Effect*. Expanded paperback ed. Cambridge: Cambridge University Press; 2009. Web. http://en.wikipedia.org/wiki/International_Standard_Book_Number

Foresight Project. *Mental Capital and Wellbeing: making the most of ourselves in the 21st century*. The Foresight Project. The Government Office for Science: London; 2008. Web.

Foucault M. *History of Madness*. London: Routledge; 2006. Print.

Fowler KA, Lilienfield SO, Patrick CJ. Detecting psychopathy from thin slices of behaviour. *Psychol Assess.* 2009; **21**: 68–78. Print.

Frackowiak RSJ, Ashburner JT, Penny WD *et al*. *Human Brain Function*. 2nd ed. San Diego, California: Academic Press; 2004. Print.

Frankel RM. From sentence to sequence: understanding the medical encounter through microinteractional analysis. *Discourse Processes.* 1984; **7**(2): 135–70. Print.

Fredrickson BL. The role of positive emotions in positive psychology: the broaden-and-build theory of positive emotions. *Am Psychol.* 2001; **56**(3): 218–26. Print.

Gabora L. The origin and evolution of culture and creativity. *Journal of Memetics.* 1997; **1**(1): n.p. Print.

Gardner, H. *Frames of Mind: The Theory of Multiple Intelligences*. 3rd ed. Basic Books, 2011. Print.

Gettier EL. Is justified true belief knowledge. *Analysis.* 1963. **23**: 121–3. Print.

Gibbs G. *Learning by Doing: a guide to teaching and learning methods.* [London]: FEU; 1988. Print.

Gilbert DT. *Stumbling on Happiness.* New York: Vintage; 2007. Print.

Gilbert E. *Eat, Pray, Love: one woman's search for everything.* New York: Penguin; 2006. Print.

Giles J. *No Self to Be Found: the search for personal identity.* Lanham: University of America; 1997. Print.

Gillon R. Medical ethics: 'four principles plus attention to scope'. *BMJ.* 1994; **309**: 184. Print.

Glaser BG, Strauss AS. *Awareness of Dying.* Chicago: Aldine Pub.; [1965]. Reprint 2005. Print.

GMC. *Disciplinary Decisions.* Rep. General Medical Council. Web. Available at: www.gmc-uk.org/concerns/hearings_and_decisions/fitness_to_practise_decisions.asp

GMC. *Good Medical Practice.* Rep. General Medical Council UK, 2006. Web. Available at: www.gmc-uk.org/guidance/good_medical_practice.asp

GMC. *Printable Documents.* Summer 2009. Web. Available at: www.gmc-uk.org/concerns/printable_documents.asp

Goldberg LR. The structure of phenotypic personality traits. *Am Psychol.* 1993; **48**: 26–34. Print.

GP Online. *A Registrar Survival Guide . . . setting up your consulting room.* GP Online. 2010. Web. Available at: www.gponline.com/Education/article/1037805/a-registrar-survival-guide-setting-consulting-room (accessed 4 November 2010).

GP Training Net. *Consultation Theory.* Web. Available at: http://gptraining.net (accessed 12 November 2011).

Grant J, Crawley J. *Transference and Projection: mirrors to the self.* Buckingham: Open University; 2002. Print.

Greene B. *The Elegant Universe: superstrings, hidden dimensions, and the quest for the ultimate theory.* London: Vintage; 2005. Print.

Greenhalgh T, Hurwitz B, editors. *Narrative Based Medicine: dialogue and discourse in clinical practice.* London: BMJ; 2002. Print.

Grimshaw GM, Stanton T. Tobacco cessation interventions for young people. *Cochrane Database Syst Rev.* 2006; **4**: CD003289. Print.

Haigh R. Modern milieux: therapeutic community solutions to acute ward problems. *The Psychiatrist.* 2002; **26**: 380–2. Print.

Haigh R. The quintessence of a therapeutic environment: five universal qualities. In: Campling P, Haigh R, editors. *Therapeutic Communities: past, present and future.* London: Jessica Kingsley; 1999. pp. 246–57. Print.

Hakeda YS. *Kukai: major works.* New York: Columbia University Press; 1972. Print.

Hall ET. *The Hidden Dimension.* Garden City, NY: Doubleday; 1966. Print.

Hammond DC. Review of the efficacy of clinical hypnosis with headaches and migraines. *IJCEH.* 2007; **55**(2): 207–19. Print.

Handy CB. *Gods of Management: the changing work of organizations.* New York: Oxford University Press; 1995. Print.

Handy CB. *Understanding Organisations.* Harmondsworth, Middlesex: Penguin; [1976] 1985. Print.

Hawking SW. *A Brief History of Time: from the big bang to black holes.* Toronto: Bantam; 1988. Print.

Health Foundation. *Evidence: helping people help themselves. A review of the evidence considering whether it is worthwhile to support self-management.* Health Foundation; May 2011. Web. Available at: www.health.org.uk/publications/evidence-helping-people-help-themselves

Health Talk Online. *Shared Decision Making.* Healthtalkonline. DOH. Web. Available at: www.healthtalkonline.org/Improving_health_care/shared_decision_making (accessed April 2011).

Hecht MA, LaFrance M. How (fast) can I help you? Tone of voice and telephone operator efficiency in interactions. *J Appl Soc Psychol.* 1995; **25**(23): 2086–98. Print.

Hélie S, Sun R. Incubation, insight, and creative problem solving: a unified theory and a connectionist model. *Psychol Rev.* 2010; **117**(3): 994–1024. Print.

Helman CG. Disease versus illness in general practice. *J R Coll Gen Pract.* 1981; **31**: 548–62. Print.

Hendrich A, Chow MP, Skierczynski BA, Lu Z. A 36-hospital time and motion study: how do medical-surgical nurses spend their time? *Perm J.* 2008; **12**(3): 25–34. Print.

Henning K, Ey S, Shaw D. Perfectionism, the impostor phenomenon and psychological adjustment in medical, dental, nursing and pharmacy students. *Med Educ.* 1998; **32**(5): 456–64. Print.

Hermans HJM, Gieser T. *Handbook of Dialogical Self Theory.* Cambridge: Cambridge University Press; 2011. Print.

Hermans HJM, Kempen HJG. *The Dialogical Self: meaning as movement.* San Diego: Academic; 1993. Print.

Heron J. A six-category intervention analysis. *Br J Guidance & Counselling.* 1976; **4**(2): 143–55. Print.

Herzberg F. *The Motivation to Work.* New York: Wiley; 1959. Print.

Hinduism Today. *Join the Hindu Renaissance.* Hinduism Today Magazine. Web. Available at: www.hinduismtoday.com (accessed 14 November 2011).

Hilbert D, Cohn-Vossen S. *Geometry and the Imagination.* 2nd ed. London: Chelsea Publishing Company; 1990. Print.

Hofstadter DR. *Gödel, Escher, Bach.* Harmondsworth: Penguin; 1980. Print.

Hume D. *A Treatise of Human Nature; being an attempt to introduce the experimental method of reasoning into moral subjects.* Cleveland: World Pub.; [1739] 1962. Print.

Hutton W. *The State We're In.* London: Jonathan Cape; 1995. Print.

Hymes J. editor. *The Child under Six.* London: Consortium; 1994. Print.

Ignatow D. *Against the Evidence: selected poems, 1934–1994.* [Middletown, Conn.]: Wesleyan University Press; 1993. Print.

Internet Encyclopedia of Philosophy. *Time.* Internet Encyclopedia of Philosophy. Web. Available at: www.iep.utm.edu/time (accessed 14 November 2011).

Isaksen SG, Treffinger DJ. *Creative Problem Solving: the basic course.* Buffalo, NY: Bearly; 1985. Print.

Isen A, Daubman KA, Nowicki GP. Positive affect facilitates creative problem solving. *J Pers Soc Psychol.* 1987; **52**(6): 1122–31. Print.

Ivancevich JM, Matteson MT. Stress and work: a managerial perspective. In: Quick JC, Bhagat RS, Dalton JE, Quick JD, editors. *Work Stress: health care systems in the workplace.* New York: Praeger; 1980. pp. 27–49. Print.

James W. *The Principles of Psychology.* Charleston, SC: BiblioLife; 2010. Print.

Juran JM, Gryna FM. *Juran's Quality Control Handbook.* New York: McGraw-Hill; 1988. Print.

Kabat-Zinn J. *Full Catastrophe Living: using the wisdom of your body and mind to face stress, pain, and illness.* New York, NY: Dell Pub., a Division of Bantam Doubleday Dell Pub. Group; 1991. Print.

Kahn RL, Byosiere P. Stress in organizations. In: Dunnette MD, Hough LM, editors. *Handbook of Industrial and Organizational Psychology, Vol. 3.* Palo Alto, CA: Consulting Psychologists Press; 1992. pp. 571–650. Print.

Kahneman D. *Thinking, Fast and Slow.* New York: Penguin; 2012. Print.

Kandel ER, Schwartz JM, Jessell TM. *Principles of Neural Science.* New York: McGraw-Hill, Health Professions Division; 2000. Print.

Kant I. *Groundwork for the Metaphysics of Morals.* New Haven: Yale University Press; 2002. Print.

Kaufman JC, Beghetto RA. Beyond big and little: the Four C Model of Creativity. *Rev Gen Psychology.* 2009; **13**: 1–12. Print.

Keating T. Centering Prayer. Web. Available at: www.centeringprayer.com (accessed 12 November 2011).

King LS. *Medical Thinking: a historical preface.* Princeton, NJ: Princeton University Press; 1982. Print.

Kleinke CL, Peterson TR, Rutledge TR. Effects of self-generated facial expressions on mood. *J Pers Soc Psychol.* 1998; **74**(1): 272–9. Print.

Kleinman A. *Patients and Healers in the Context of Culture: an exploration of the borderland between anthropology, medicine, and psychiatry.* Berkeley: University of California; 1980. Print.

Ko U. Ananda. *Beyond Self: 108 Korean Zen poems.* Berkeley, CA: Parallax; 1997. Print.

Koch R. *The Natural Laws of Business: applying the theories of Darwin, Einstein, and Newton to achieve business success.* New York: Currency/Doubleday; 2001. Print.

Koestler A. *The Ghost in the Machine.* London: Hutchinson; 1967. Print.

Kolb DA. *Experiential Learning: experience as the source of learning and development.* Englewood Cliffs, NJ: Prentice-Hall; 1984. Print.

Kornfield J. *Buddha's Little Instruction Book.* London: Rider & Co; 1996. Print.

Kotter JP. *Leading Change.* Boston, MA: Harvard Business School; 1996. Print.

Kumar M. *Quantum: Einstein, Bohr, and the great debate about the nature of reality.* New York: W.W. Norton; 2009. Print.

Kurtz SM, Silverman J, Draper J. *Teaching and Learning Communication Skills in Medicine.* Oxford: Radcliffe Publishing; 2005. Print.

Lalor D. *Creating a Therapeutic Environment. Counselling in Perth, Western Australia.* Cottesloe Counselling Centre. Web. Available at: www.cottesloecounselling.com.au (accessed 24 October 2011).

Lazarus RS, Folkman S. *Stress, Appraisal, and Coping.* New York: Springer; 1984.

Launer J. *Narrative-based Primary Care: a practical guide*. Oxford: Radcliffe Medical Press; 2002. Print.

Légaré F, Ratté S, Stacey D, *et al*. Interventions for improving the adoption of shared decision making by healthcare professionals. *Cochrane Database Syst Rev*. 2011; **10**: CD001431. Web.

Lehrer J. *Imagine: how creativity works*. Edinburgh: Canongate; 2012. Print.

Levensky E, Forcehimes A, Beitz K. Motivational interviewing: an evidence-based approach to counseling helps patients follow treatment recommendations. *Am J Nurs*. 2007; **107**(10): 50–8. Print.

Lewin S, Skea Z, Entwistle V, *et al*. Effects of interventions to promote a patient-centred approach in clinical consultations. *Cochrane Database Syst Rev*. 2001; **4**: CD00326. Web.

Lewin SA, Skea Z, Entwistle VA, *et al*. Interventions for providers to promote a patient-centred approach in clinical consultations. *Cochrane Database Syst Rev*. 2012; **12**: CD003267. Print.

Linehan M. *Cognitive Behavioural Treatment of Borderline Personality Disorder*. London: Guildford; 1993. Print.

Linn LS, Yager J, Cope D, Leake B. Health status, job satisfaction, job stress, and life satisfaction among academic and clinical faculty. *JAMA*. 1985; **254**(19): 2775–82. Print.

Living Life to the Full. *Free Online Skills Course*. Living Life to the Full. Web. Available at: www.llttf.com (accessed 28 October 2011).

Locke J, Bassett T, Holt E. *An Essay Concerning Humane Understanding: in four books*. London: Printed by Eliz. Holt for Thomas Basset; 1690. Print.

Mackenzie RA. *The Time Trap*. New York: AMACOM; 1972. Print.

Maslach C, Schaufeli W, Leiter M. Job burnout. *Annu Rev Psychol*. 2001; **52**: 397–422. Web.

Maslow AH. A theory of human motivation. *Psychol Rev*. 1943; **50**(4): 370–96. Print.

Maslow AH. *The Farther Reaches of Human Nature*. New York: Penguin; 1976. Print.

May R. *The Courage to Create*. London: Collins; 1976. Print.

McCambridge J. Motivational interviewing is equivalent to more intensive treatment, superior to placebo, and will be tested more widely. *Evidence-Based Mental Health*. 2004. **7**(2): 52. Print.

McKinlay JB, Potter DA, Feldman DA. Non-medical influences on medical decision-making. *Soc Sci Med*. 1996; **42**(5): 769–76. Print.

McQuaid JR, Carmona PE. *Peaceful Mind: using mindfulness and cognitive behavioral psychology to overcome depression*. Oakland, CA: New Harbinger; 2004. Print.

McVicar A. Workplace stress in nursing: a literature review. *J Adv Nurs*. 2003; **44**(6): 633–42. Print.

Melville A. Job satisfaction in general practice: implications for prescribing. *Soc Sci Med. Part A: Medical Psychology & Medical Sociology*. 1980; **14**(6): 495–9. Print.

Mitchley SE. The medical interview: the three-function approach. *Postgrad Med J*. 1992; **68**(799): 397–8. Print.

MoodGYM. Welcome. Web. Available at: www.moodgym.anu.edu.au (accessed 28 October 2011).

Moran P. *Antisocial Personality Disorder*. London: Gaskell; 1999. Print.

Morrison T. *Staff Supervision in Social Care: making a real difference for staff and service users*. Brighton: Pavilion; 2005. Print.

National Institute for Health and Care Excellence. *Anxiety: management of anxiety (panic disorder, with or without agoraphobia, and generalised anxiety disorder) in adults in primary, secondary and community care*. NICE. March 2011. Web. Available at: http://guidance.nice.org.uk/CG22

National Institute for Health and Care Excellence. *Brief Interventions and Referral for Smoking Cessation in Primary Care and Other Settings*. NICE. 2006. Web. Available at: www.nice.org.uk/nicemedia/pdf/SMOKING-ALS2_FINAL.pdf

National Institute for Health and Care Excellence. *Cognitive Behavioural Therapy for the Management of Common Mental Health Problems*. NICE. December 2010. Web. Available at: www.nice.org.uk/usingguidance/commissioningguides/cognitivebehavioural therapyservice/cbt.jsp

National Institute for Health and Care Excellence. *Computerised Cognitive Behaviour Therapy for Depression and Anxiety: review of Technology Appraisal 51*. NICE. February 2006. Web. Available at: www.nice.org.uk/nicemedia/pdf/TA097guidance.pdf

Neighbour R. *The Inner Consultation: how to develop an effective and intuitive consulting style*. Lancaster: MTP; 1987. Print.

NHS Centre for Reviews. *Effectiveness Matters: counselling in primary care*. 2001; **5**(2): n.p. Print.

NHS Direct. *Decision Aids*. NHS Direct. Web. Available at: www.nhsdirect.nhs.uk/decisionaids.

NHS Institute for Innovation and Improvement. *Releasing Time to Care: the productive ward*. 2007. Available at: www.institute.nhs.uk/quality_and_value/productivity_series/productive_ward.html.

Noonuccal, Oodgeroo. *My People*. 3rd ed. Milton, QA: The Jacaranda Press; 1990. Print.

Ogedegbe G. Labeling and hypertension: it is time to intervene on its negative consequences. *Hypertension*. 2010; **56**(3): 344–5. Print.

O'Hara LA. Creativity and intelligence. In: Sternberg RJ, editor. *Handbook of Creativity*. Cambridge University Press; 1999. Print.

Open Door Coaching. *Job Satisfaction Inventory*. Open Door Coaching. Web. Available at: www.opendoorcoaching.com/PDF%20files/Job%20Satisfaction%20Inventory.PDF (accessed 24 October 2011).

Orwell G. *Nineteen Eighty-four, a novel*. New York: Harcourt, Brace; 1949. Print.

'Overcoming' series. Constable & Robinson Publishers. Web. Available at: www.overcoming.co.uk

Paice E, Moss F. How important are role models in making good doctors. *BMJ*. 2002; **325**: 707. Print.

Patient.co.uk. *Significant Event Analysis*. Health Information and Advice, Medicines Guide, Patient.co.uk. Web. Available at: http://patient.co.uk (accessed 24 October 2011).

Patrick CJ, Craig KD, Prkachin KM. Observer judgments of acute pain: facial action determinants. *J Pers Soc Psych*. 1986; **50**(6): 1291–8. Print.

Pendleton D, Schofield T, Tate P, Havelock P. *The Consultation: an approach to learning and teaching*. Oxford: Oxford University Press; 1984. Print.

Penrose R. *The Emperor's New Mind: concerning computers, minds, and the laws of physics*. Oxford: Oxford University Press; 1989. Print.

Pepler D J. Play and divergent thinking. In: Pepler DJ, Rubin KH. *The Play of Children: current theory and research*. Basel; New York: Karger; 1982. Print.

Pepler DJ, Rubin KH, editors. *The Play of Children: current theory and research*. Basel; New York: Karger; 1982. Print.

Prkachin KM. Dissociating spontaneous and deliberate expressions of pain: signal detection analyses. *Pain*. 1992; **51**(1): 57–65. Print.

Prochaska JO, DiClemente CC. *The Transtheoretical Approach: crossing traditional boundaries of therapy*. Malabar, Florida: R. E. Krieger; 1994. Print.

Proshansky H. The field of environmental psychology. *Handbook of Environmental Psychology*. New York: Wiley; 1987. Print.

Proshansky H, Fabian A, Kaminoff R. Place-identity: physical world socialization of the self. *J Environ Psychol*. 1983; **3**(1): 57–83. Print.

Quakers. *Quaker Faith & Practice: the book of Christian discipline of the yearly meeting of the Religious Society of Friends (Quakers) in Britain*. London: Yearly Meeting of the Religious Society of Friends (Quakers) in Britain; 2009. Print.

Reuler JB, Nardone DA. Role modeling in medical education. *West J Med*. 1994; **160**(4): 335–7. Print.

Rolfe G, Freshwater D, Jasper M. *Critical Reflection for Nursing and the Helping Professions: a user's guide*. Houndmills, Basingstoke, Hampshire: Palgrave; 2001. Print.

Rossman J. *Industrial Creativity; the psychology of the inventor*. New Hyde Park, NY: University; 1964. Print.

Roter DL, Frankel RM, Hall JA, Sluyter D. The expression of emotion through nonverbal behavior in medical visits. Mechanisms and outcomes. *J Gen Intern Med*. 2006; **21**(Suppl. 1): S28–34. Print.

Sackett DL, Rosenberg WM, Gray JA, *et al*. Evidence based medicine: what it is and what it isn't. *BMJ*. 1996; **312**: 71–2. Print.

Sandman, L, Munthe C. Shared decision making, paternalism and patient choice. *Health Care Anal*. 2010; **18**(1): 60–84. Print.

Schegloff EA, Jefferson G, Sacks H. The preference for self-correction in the organization of repair in conversation. *Language*. 1977; **53**: 361–82. Print.

Schön DA. *The Reflective Practitioner: how professionals think in action*. Aldershot: Ashgate; [1983] 2002. Print.

Schwarz, B. *The Paradox of Choice: why more is less*. HarperCollins; New edition; 2005. Print.

Searle JR. *Mind: a brief introduction*. Oxford: Oxford University Press; 2004. Print.

Segal Z, Williams JM, Teasdale J. *Mindfulness-Based Cognitive Therapy for Depression: a new approach to preventing relapse*. New York: Guildford; 2001. Print.

Seligman MEP. *Authentic Happiness: using the new positive psychology to realize your potential for lasting fulfillment*. New York: Free; 2002. Print.

Sharot T, De Martino B, Dolan RJ. Neural activity predicts attitude change in cognitive dissonance. *Nature Neuroscience*. 2009; **29**(12): 3760–5. Print.

Silverman J, Kurtz SM, Draper J. *Skills for Communicating with Patients*. 3rd ed. London: Radcliffe Publishing; 2013. Print.

Simon HA. The mind's eye in chess. In: Chase WG, editor. *Visual Information Processing*. New York: Academic; 1973. Print.

Simon P, Garfunkel A. *The Sounds of Silence*. Columbia, released 1965. CD.

Simonton DK. Creativity, leadership, and chance. In: Sternberg RJ, editor. *The Nature of Creativity*. Cambridge: Cambridge University Press; 1988. Print.

Smith HW. *The 10 Natural Laws of Successful Time and Life Management: proven strategies for increased productivity and inner peace*. New York, NY: Warner; 2003. Print.

Snyder CR, Lopez SJ, editors. *Handbook of Positive Psychology*. Oxford: Oxford University Press; 2009. Print.

Soria R, Legido A, Escolano C. A randomised controlled trial of motivational interviewing for smoking cessation. *Br J Gen Pract*. 2006; **1**(56): 531. Print.

Sowa JF. 'Representing knowledge soup in language and logic'. Available online at: www.jfsowa.com/talks/souprepr.htm

Sternberg RJ. *Beyond IQ: A Triarchic Theory of Intelligence*. Cambridge: Cambridge University Press; 1985.

Stewart I, Joines V. *TA Today: a new introduction to transactional analysis*. Nottingham: Lifespace Pub.; 1987. Print.

Stewart M, Roter D. *Communicating with Medical Patients*. Newbury Park: Sage Publications; 1989. Print.

Stiglitz JE, Sen A, Fitoussi J-P. *Report by the Commission on the Measurement of Economic Performance and Social Progress*. Paris: Commission; 2009. Print.

Stott NC, Davis RH. The exceptional potential in each primary care consultation. *J R Coll Gen Pract*. 1979; **29**: 201–5. Print.

Suzuki DT. *Essays in Zen Buddhism, third series*. London: Published for the Buddhist Society by Rider; 1958. Print.

Suzuki S, Dixon T. *Zen Mind, Beginner's Mind*. New York: Walker/Weatherhill; 1970. Print.

Tarski A. *Logic, Semantics, Metamathematics; papers from 1923 to 1938*. Oxford: Clarendon; 1956. Print.

Taylor D, Bury M. Chronic illness, expert patients and care transition. *Sociology of Health & Illness*. 2007; **29**(1): 27–45. Print.

Tellegen A, Lykken DT, Bouchard TJ, *et al.* Personality similarity in twins reared apart and together. *J Pers Soc Psychol*. 1988; **54**(6): 1031–9. Print.

Thich Nhat Hanh, Mobi Ho, Vo-Dinh Mai. *Miracle of Mindfulness: an introduction*. Boston: Beacon; 1975. Print.

Top Nursing Colleges. *Nursing Theories and Sub-theories*. Top Nursing Colleges. Web. Available at: www.topnursingcolleges.com/nur/nursing-theories-and-sub-theories.html (accessed 12 November 2011).

Tsao L. How much do we know about the importance of play in child development. *Childhood Educ*. Summer 2002. Findarticles.com. Web. Available at: http://findarticles.com/p/articles/mi_qa3614/is_200207/ai_n9147500

Tuckett D, Boulton M, Olson C, Williams A. *Meetings between Experts: an approach to sharing ideas in medical consultations*. London: Tavistock, 1985. Print.

Ubel PA, Angott AM, Zikmund-Fischer BJ. Physicians recommend different treatment for patients than they would choose for themselves. *Arch Intern Med*. 2011; **171**(18): 630–4. Print.

Ulrich RS. How design impacts wellness. *Healthc Forum J.* 1992; **35**(5): 20–5. Print.

Upton J. *Comments*. FearFighter for Panic and Anxiety. Web. Available at: www.fear fighter.com (accessed 28 October 2011).

US National Cancer Institute. *Cancer Screening Overview (PDQ®)*. US National Cancer Institute. Web. Available at: www.cancer.gov/cancertopics/pdq/screening/overview/HealthProfessional/page1 (accessed 24 October 2011).

Van Ham I, Verhoeven A, Groenier K, Groothoff J and De Haan J. Job satisfaction among general practitioners: A systematic literature review. *Eur J Gen Pract.* 2006, **12**(4): 174–80. (doi:10.1080/13814780600994376)

Van Veen V, Krug MK, Scooler JW, Carter CS. Neural activity predicts attitude change in cognitive dissonance. *Nature Neuroscience.* 2009; **12**(11): 1469–74. Print.

Vandervert L, Schimpf P, Liu H. How working memory and the cerebellum collaborate to produce creativity and innovation. *Creativity Res J.* 2007; **19**(1): 1–18. Print.

Various. Evidence based practice in clinical hypnosis. *IJCEH.* 2007; **55**(2): n.p. Print.

Walker L. *Consulting with NLP: Neuro-linguistic Programming in the medical consultation*. Oxford: Radcliffe Medical Press; 2002. Print.

Wallas G. *The Art of Thought*. New York: Harcourt, Brace; 1926. Print.

Warren KS. *Coping with the Biomedical Literature: a primer for the scientist and the clinician*. New York, NY: Praeger; 1981. Print.

Waskett C. An integrated approach to introducing and maintaining supervision: the 4S Model. *Nurs Times.* 2009; **105**(17): 24–6. Print.

Weisberg RW. *Creativity: beyond the myth of genius*. New York: W.H. Freeman; 1993. Print.

West C. Against our will: male interruptions of females in cross-sex conversation. *Annals of the New York Academy of Sciences.* 1979 (Language, Sex); **327**(1): 81–96. Print.

White M. *Maps of Narrative Practice*. New York: W.W. Norton & Co; 2007. Print.

White M, Epston D. *Narrative Means to Therapeutic Ends*. New York: Norton; 1990. Print.

Wilber K. *A Brief History of Everything*. Boston, MA: Shambhala; 2007. Print.

Wilber K. An integral theory of consciousness. *J Consciousness Stud.* 1997; **4**(1): 71–92. Print.

Williams CJ, Garland A. Cognitive-behavioural therapy assessment model for use in clinical practice. *Adv Psych Treat.* 2002; **8**: 172–79. Print.

Williams ES, Konrad TR. Physician, practice, and patient characteristics related to primary care physician physical and mental health: results from the Physician Worklife Study. *Health Services Res.* 2002; **37**(1): 119–41. Print.

Williams ES, Konrad TR, Scheckler WE, *et al*. Understanding physicians' intentions to withdraw from practice: the role of job satisfaction, job stress, mental and physical health. *Health Care Manage Rev.* 2010; **35**(2): 105–15. Web.

Wilson PM, Kendall S, Brooks F. The Expert Patients Programme: a paradox of patient empowerment and medical dominance. *Health & Social Care in the Community.* 2007; **15**(5): 426–38. Web.

Yovel G, Kanwisher N. Face perception: domain specific, not process specific. *Neuron.* 2004; **44**(5): 889–98. Print.

Zhong E, Kenward K, Sheets V, *et al*. Probation and recidivism: remediation among disciplined nurses in six states. *Am J Nurs.* 2009; **109**(3): 48–57. Print.

CPD with Radcliffe

You can now use a selection of our books to achieve CPD (Continuing Professional Development) points through directed reading.

We provide a free online form and downloadable certificate for your appraisal portfolio. Look for the CPD logo and register with us at: www.radcliffehealth.com/cpd

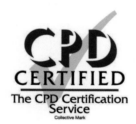